HEMODYNAMIC MONITORING MADE EASY: MASTERING CRITICAL CARE SKILLS FOR NURSES AND CLINICIANS

By

Dr. Joan HAMPTON

Table of Contents

Introduction

- **Welcome to Hemodynamic Monitoring**
- Why This Guide is Important
- Who This Book is For
- Overview of Hemodynamics: From Basics to Bedside

Chapter 1: Hemodynamics Made Easy

- Understanding the Cardiovascular System
- Key Terminology: Preload, Afterload, Cardiac Output, Stroke Volume
- The Role of Hemodynamic Monitoring in Critical Care

Chapter 2: Tools of the Trade

- Overview of Monitoring Equipment
- Setting Up and Calibrating Equipment Safely
- Troubleshooting Common Equipment Issues
- Maintaining Sterility and Minimizing Infections

Chapter 3: Core Hemodynamic Parameters Explained

- Central Venous Pressure (CVP)
- Mean Arterial Pressure (MAP)
- Cardiac Output (CO) and Cardiac Index (CI)
- Pulmonary Capillary Wedge Pressure (PCWP)
- Systemic and Pulmonary Vascular Resistance (SVR and PVR)

Chapter 4: Hemodynamic Waveform Analysis

- Understanding Pressure Waveforms
- Arterial, Venous, and Pulmonary Artery Pressure Waves
- Recognizing Normal vs. Abnormal Waveforms
- Troubleshooting Artifacts and Abnormalities

Chapter 5: Step-by-Step Guide to Invasive Hemodynamic Monitoring

- Insertion and Management of Arterial Lines
- Central Venous Catheters: Placement and Management
- Pulmonary Artery Catheterization Techniques
- Dynamic Assessments: Passive Leg Raise, Fluid Challenge

Chapter 6: Non-Invasive Hemodynamic Monitoring

- Doppler Ultrasound and Echocardiography
- Pulse Contour Analysis
- Advanced Non-Invasive Techniques

Chapter 7: Hemodynamic Assessment for Different Clinical Scenarios

- Managing Hypotension and Shock
- Hemodynamic Changes in Sepsis and Cardiogenic Shock
- Monitoring in Patients with Heart Failure
- Hemodynamic Considerations in Post-Operative Care

Chapter 8: Fluid Management and Volume Resuscitation

- Assessing Fluid Status Using Hemodynamic Parameters
- Fluid Challenge: When and How
- Volume Overload: Detection and Management

Chapter 9: Pharmacology for Hemodynamic Management

- Inotropes, Vasopressors, and Vasodilators Explained
- Pharmacologic Interventions for Common Hemodynamic Issues
- Drug Dosing Considerations and Side Effects

Chapter 10: Hemodynamic Case Studies and Clinical Application

- Real-World Case Studies: From Simple to Complex
- Critical Thinking and Decision-Making Pathways
- Common Pitfalls and How to Avoid Them

Chapter 11: Quick Reference Guides and Cheat Sheets

- Normal Hemodynamic Values and Ranges
- Quick Troubleshooting for Equipment Issues
- Medication Dosing Charts for Hemodynamic Agents

Chapter 12: Frequently Asked Questions

- Addressing Common Concerns and Misconceptions
- Expert Tips for Beginners in Hemodynamic Monitoring

Conclusion

- Summary of Key Concepts
- Additional Resources for Continued Learning
- How to Apply What You've Learned to Real-World Practice

Appendices

- **Appendix A**: Hemodynamic Monitoring Checklist
- **Appendix B**: Hemodynamic Formulas and Calculations
- **Appendix C**: Glossary of Hemodynamic Terms

THE END

INTRODUCTION

Hemodynamic monitoring is a cornerstone of modern critical care, providing invaluable insights into a patient's cardiovascular status and guiding life-saving interventions. For clinicians, understanding the principles of hemodynamics is not just a skill but a critical competency that directly impacts patient outcomes. Yet, mastering these principles can seem daunting, especially for beginners.

This book is designed to demystify the complexities of hemodynamic monitoring and empower you, whether you're a nurse, physician, or clinical staff, to confidently apply these concepts in real-world settings. We've structured the content to build from foundational knowledge to more advanced clinical applications, ensuring a smooth learning curve. Throughout, we focus on practical insights, case studies, and clear explanations to help translate theoretical knowledge into actionable skills.

While you're new to healthcare or trying to improve your skills, this guide provides step-by-step instructions, visual aids, and clinical pearls to help you better comprehend cardiovascular dynamics. By the end of this book, you'll be proficient in setting up and interpreting hemodynamic monitors and skilled at making informed clinical decisions that could make the difference between life and death.

So, why is this guide important, and who is it for? Let's go into these questions to provide the groundwork for what comes next.

WHY THIS GUIDE IS IMPORTANT

Hemodynamic monitoring is crucial for various reasons:

1. Early Detection of Complications: Continuous monitoring of cardiovascular parameters allows clinicians to identify complications such as shock, heart failure, and fluid imbalances early, providing a window for timely interventions.

2. Personalized Patient Care: By accurately assessing a patient's hemodynamic status, clinicians can tailor treatments such as fluid management, medication adjustments, and mechanical support, improving patient outcomes.

3. Preventing Treatment Errors: Misinterpretation of hemodynamic data can lead to inappropriate treatment decisions, potentially worsening a patient's condition. This guide will help you avoid common pitfalls and enhance your confidence in making informed clinical choices.

4. Building a Strong Clinical Foundation: For healthcare professionals, mastering hemodynamic monitoring lays a solid foundation for understanding other advanced cardiovascular topics. It is a stepping stone toward more complex skills such as echocardiography and advanced life support.

We understand that the initial learning curve can be steep. That's why this book takes a step-by-step approach, making the journey from novice to expert achievable and rewarding.

WHO THIS BOOK IS FOR

This book is suitable for:

- **Nurses and Clinical Staff:** New graduates or those transitioning into critical care settings will find this guide invaluable in gaining confidence and competence in hemodynamic monitoring.
- **Medical Students and Residents:** It serves as a foundational text for understanding cardiovascular physiology and applying hemodynamic principles in clinical practice.
- **Experienced Practitioners:** For those looking to refresh their knowledge or expand into more advanced techniques, this book covers both basic and complex topics, providing a comprehensive review.
- **Critical Care Teams:** Multidisciplinary teams including physicians, nurse practitioners, and physician assistants can use this book to standardize hemodynamic monitoring practices and optimize patient care.

OVERVIEW OF HEMODYNAMICS: FROM BASICS TO BEDSIDE

The term **hemodynamics** refers to the study of blood flow and its properties as it circulates through the cardiovascular system. It encompasses key parameters such as blood pressure, cardiac output, vascular resistance, and oxygen delivery. Understanding these parameters is essential for evaluating a patient's cardiovascular status and identifying any abnormalities.

In clinical practice, hemodynamic monitoring serves several purposes:

- **Assessing Cardiac Function:** Helps in determining how effectively the heart is pumping and whether cardiac output is sufficient to meet the body's needs.
- **Guiding Therapeutic Interventions:** Hemodynamic data guides the use of fluids, medications, and mechanical support (e.g., ventilators or intra-aortic balloon pumps) to stabilize patients.
- **Monitoring Response to Treatmen**t: Continuous or periodic monitoring enables clinicians to assess how well a patient is responding to interventions, allowing for real-time adjustments.

This guide will walk you through the various aspects of hemodynamic monitoring, starting from basic concepts like preload, afterload, and contractility, to more advanced topics such as waveform analysis and pharmacological management. You'll learn not only how to collect and analyze data, but also how to think critically about what these figures indicate for your patient's care.

By the end of this book, you'll be equipped to confidently approach any clinical scenario involving hemodynamic monitoring, regardless of whether it is managing a patient in shock, improving cardiac output in heart failure, or fine-tuning fluid management post-surgery.

Now that we've set the foundation, let's explain deeply into the core concepts of hemodynamics, starting with an easy-to-understand breakdown of the basic principles.

CHAPTER ONE

Hemodynamics Made Easy

Hemodynamics refers to the dynamics of blood flow and the forces that influence its circulation throughout the body. Understanding hemodynamics is fundamental to delivering effective care in critically ill patients, where rapid changes in cardiovascular status can lead to life-threatening conditions. However, hemodynamics is often perceived as a complex topic, filled with intricate physiological relationships and daunting clinical measurements. This chapter aims to simplify these complexities, making the core principles easy to grasp and clinically applicable.

In this chapter, we'll begin by breaking down the anatomy and function of the cardiovascular system, highlighting how blood moves through the heart, vessels, and organs. We'll then explore key terms like **preload**, **afterload**, **cardiac output**, and **stroke volume**—the building blocks of hemodynamic understanding. These terms are essential for interpreting patient status and making sound clinical decisions.

Finally, we'll go into the pivotal role hemodynamic monitoring plays in critical care settings, where accurate measurements and interpretations can guide interventions that stabilize patients and save lives. Whether you're a novice seeking foundational knowledge or a seasoned clinician wanting to brush up on the basics, this chapter will equip you with a solid understanding of hemodynamic principles.

Let's start by reviewing the structure and function of the cardiovascular system, which forms the basis for everything else in hemodynamics.

UNDERSTANDING THE CARDIOVASCULAR SYSTEM

To effectively interpret hemodynamic data and make informed clinical decisions, it's essential to first have a solid understanding of the cardiovascular system and how it functions. The cardiovascular system, also known as the circulatory system, is a complex network of the heart, blood vessels, and blood that works to deliver oxygen, nutrients, and hormones to tissues and organs while also removing waste products like carbon dioxide.

The Structure of the Cardiovascular System

The cardiovascular system can be divided into three major components:

1. **The Heart**: The heart is a muscular organ that acts as the pump of the cardiovascular system, ensuring continuous blood flow throughout the body. It is divided into four chambers:
   - **Right Atrium**: Receives deoxygenated blood from the body via the superior and inferior vena cava.
   - **Right Ventricle**: Pumps deoxygenated blood to the lungs through the pulmonary artery for oxygenation.
   - **Left Atrium**: Receives oxygenated blood from the lungs via the pulmonary veins.
   - **Left Ventricle**: Pumps oxygenated blood to the entire body through the aorta, generating systemic circulation.
2. Each chamber is separated by valves—tricuspid, pulmonary, mitral, and aortic—that ensure unidirectional blood flow and prevent backflow. The left ventricle has the thickest muscular wall because it needs to generate high pressure to propel blood through systemic circulation.
3. **The Blood Vessels**: Blood vessels are classified into arteries, veins, and capillaries, each with a distinct role:
   - **Arteries**: Thick-walled vessels that carry oxygen-rich blood away from the heart to the tissues. The aorta is the

largest artery.
- **Veins**: Thin-walled vessels that carry deoxygenated blood back to the heart. They have valves to prevent blood from pooling or flowing backward.
- **Capillaries**: Tiny blood vessels that connect arteries and veins, facilitating the exchange of oxygen, nutrients, and waste products between blood and tissues.
4. **The Blood**: Blood is the transport medium, composed of red blood cells (carry oxygen), white blood cells (immune function), platelets (clotting), and plasma (fluid containing proteins, nutrients, and waste products).

How Blood Circulates: The Two Circuits

The cardiovascular system operates in two major circuits:

1. **Pulmonary Circulation**: Involves the movement of blood from the heart to the lungs and back. The right ventricle pumps deoxygenated blood to the lungs via the pulmonary artery. In the lungs, carbon dioxide is exchanged for oxygen. The oxygenated blood then returns to the left atrium via the pulmonary veins.
2. **Systemic Circulation**: This is the larger of the two circuits and involves the movement of oxygen-rich blood from the left ventricle to the body's tissues. Once oxygen is delivered and waste products are collected, the deoxygenated blood returns to the right atrium via the superior and inferior vena cava.

Understanding Blood Flow and Pressure

Blood flow is driven by pressure differences created by the heart's pumping action. The higher the pressure gradient, the greater the flow. Blood pressure is highest in the arteries and decreases as it moves through the arterioles, capillaries, and veins. This pressure gradient is crucial for ensuring effective tissue perfusion.

In clinical practice, it's essential to assess not just blood flow but also how well the heart is functioning as a pump and whether the blood vessels are adequately maintaining pressure. This is where hemodynamic monitoring comes into play, allowing you to measure parameters like cardiac output, blood pressure, and vascular resistance.

The Cardiac Cycle: Systole and Diastole

The cardiac cycle consists of two main phases:

1. **Systole**: This is the contraction phase, where the ventricles pump blood out of the heart. During systole:
   - The right ventricle sends blood to the lungs.
   - The left ventricle pumps blood to the rest of the body.
2. **Diastole**: This is the relaxation phase, where the ventricles fill with blood. It is essential for adequate preload, which refers to the volume of blood in the ventricles at the end of diastole, just before the heart contracts again.

Both phases are crucial to maintaining proper cardiac function and systemic circulation. Any disruption in the balance between systole and diastole can lead to hemodynamic instability, which can be detected through monitoring techniques.

The Heart as a Pump: Measuring Its Effectiveness

The heart's effectiveness as a pump is determined by several factors, including:

- **Heart Rate (HR)**: The number of times the heart beats per minute.
- **Stroke Volume (SV)**: The amount of blood ejected by each ventricle during systole.
- **Cardiac Output (CO)**: The total volume of blood the heart pumps per minute, calculated as CO = HR × SV.

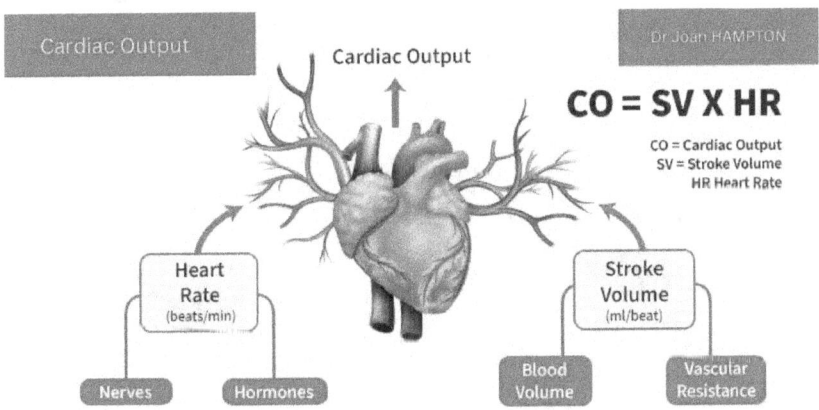

Fig 1.0: Cardiac Output

Understanding these variables is crucial for hemodynamic monitoring because they reflect the overall function of the heart and its ability to meet the body's demands. Variations in heart rate, stroke volume, and cardiac output can indicate underlying cardiovascular conditions, necessitating prompt intervention.

A solid understanding of the cardiovascular system's structure and function is the foundation of hemodynamics. From the heart's chambers and valves to the vast network of vessels, every component plays a critical role in ensuring effective circulation. By grasping how these elements interact, you'll be better equipped to interpret hemodynamic data, recognize abnormalities, and implement appropriate clinical actions.

With this foundational understanding in place, let's define crucial concepts such as preload, afterload, cardiac output, and stroke volume —terms you'll see throughout this book.

KEY TERMINOLOGY: PRELOAD, AFTERLOAD, CARDIAC OUTPUT, STROKE VOLUME

In the field of hemodynamic monitoring, a clear understanding of certain core terms is essential for interpreting patient status and guiding interventions. Terms like **preload, afterload, cardiac output**, and **stroke volume** are the foundation of cardiovascular physiology and help clinicians evaluate the heart's efficiency as a pump. Let's break down these critical concepts:

1. Preload: The Heart's Volume Load

Preload refers to the degree of stretch in the cardiac muscle fibers at the end of diastole, right before the heart contracts. In simple terms, it's the volume of blood filling the ventricles just before the next heartbeat. Preload is influenced by the amount of blood returning to the heart (venous return) and the compliance (stretchability) of the ventricle walls.

- **Key Points**:
    1. Preload is often described as the "filling pressure" of the heart.
    2. It is proportional to the end-diastolic volume (EDV) of the ventricles.
    3. An increase in venous return will elevate preload, whereas a decrease in venous return (e.g., due to hemorrhage or dehydration) will lower preload.
- **Why Preload Matters in Hemodynamic Monitoring**: Preload is a critical determinant of cardiac output, according to the **Frank-Starling law**. This principle states that the more the heart is filled (increased preload), the stronger the force of contraction will be, up to an optimal point. This is crucial in assessing fluid

status and optimizing fluid resuscitation in critically ill patients.
- **Clinical Measurement**: Preload can be indirectly assessed using parameters such as **central venous pressure (CVP)** and **pulmonary capillary wedge pressure (PCWP)**. However, these measurements should be interpreted cautiously as they are affected by many factors beyond preload alone.
- **Illustrative Table Idea**: Include a table illustrating various factors that increase and decrease preload, such as patient positioning, venous tone, and intrathoracic pressure.

2. Afterload: The Resistance to Pumping

Afterload is the resistance or pressure that the heart must overcome to eject blood during systole. Imagine afterload as the "weight" against which the heart is pushing blood out of the ventricles. It is determined by the diameter and elasticity of blood vessels, blood viscosity, and overall vascular resistance.

- **Key Points**:
    1. Afterload is influenced by systemic vascular resistance (SVR) and pulmonary vascular resistance (PVR).
    2. A high afterload (e.g., due to hypertension or aortic stenosis) makes it harder for the heart to pump blood, increasing the workload on the ventricles.
    3. A low afterload (e.g., due to vasodilation) reduces the force needed to pump blood, making it easier for the heart.
- **Why Afterload Matters in Hemodynamic Monitoring**: Afterload has a direct impact on stroke volume and cardiac output. An increase in afterload can lead to a decrease in stroke volume if the heart is unable to generate enough force to overcome it. This is crucial in managing conditions like heart failure and hypertension.
- **Clinical Measurement**: Afterload is commonly evaluated using parameters such as **systemic vascular resistance (SVR)** and **mean arterial pressure (MAP)**. It can also be affected by changes in intravascular volume and medications like vasodilators or vasoconstrictors.
- **Suggested Chart Idea**: Include a bar chart comparing normal SVR and MAP values with those seen in conditions of high and low afterload, to visually demonstrate how changes in

resistance affect the heart.

3. Cardiac Output (CO): The Heart's Pumping Capacity

Cardiac output is the total volume of blood ejected by the heart per minute. It is a key indicator of the heart's efficiency and the body's perfusion status. Cardiac output is calculated as the product of heart rate and stroke volume:

Cardiac Output (CO)=Heart Rate (HR)×Stroke Volume (SV)

- **Key Points**:
    1. The normal range for cardiac output is 4–8 liters per minute.
    2. A high cardiac output indicates increased tissue perfusion, often seen in hypermetabolic states or sepsis.
    3. A low cardiac output suggests reduced tissue perfusion, common in heart failure or hypovolemia.
- **Why Cardiac Output Matters in Hemodynamic Monitoring**: Cardiac output reflects the overall function of the cardiovascular system and whether the body's tissues are receiving adequate oxygen and nutrients. It is a critical parameter in assessing patient stability and guiding interventions like fluid therapy or inotropic support.
- **Clinical Measurement**: Cardiac output can be measured using thermodilution techniques via a pulmonary artery catheter, Doppler ultrasound, or newer non-invasive technologies. In some settings, **cardiac index (CI)** is used, which is CO adjusted for body surface area (BSA).
- **Illustrative Diagram Idea**: Include a flowchart demonstrating the relationship between heart rate, stroke volume, and factors that increase or decrease each, giving a holistic view of what influences cardiac output.

4. Stroke Volume (SV): The Heart's Ejection Per Beat

Stroke volume is the amount of blood ejected by the left ventricle with each heartbeat. It's a key component of cardiac output and is influenced by preload, afterload, and myocardial contractility.

- **Key Points**:
    1. The normal range for stroke volume is approximately 60–100 mL per beat.

2. Stroke volume is directly proportional to preload and contractility and inversely proportional to afterload.
3. Decreased stroke volume can result from conditions like myocardial infarction, fluid loss, or increased afterload.

- **Why Stroke Volume Matters in Hemodynamic Monitoring**: Stroke volume is a more specific indicator of left ventricular function compared to heart rate. Monitoring changes in stroke volume helps identify the cause of decreased cardiac output and guides targeted interventions.
- **Clinical Measurement**: Stroke volume can be calculated using echocardiography or advanced hemodynamic monitoring systems that estimate parameters like stroke volume variation (SVV).

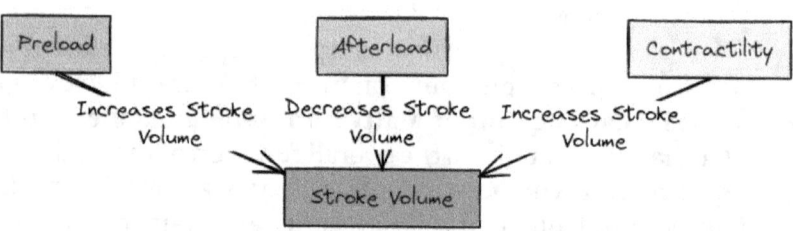

Fig 1.1: Relationship between preload, afterload, and contractility, and how they collectively influence stroke volume

Understanding preload, afterload, cardiac output, and stroke volume is critical for hemodynamic monitoring. These factors are interconnected and provide information about the heart's efficiency as a pump, the resistance it encounters, and the general condition of a patient's circulation. By grasping these fundamental concepts, clinicians may enhance patient care, personalize interventions, and improve outcomes in crucial situations.

THE ROLE OF HEMODYNAMIC MONITORING IN CRITICAL CARE

Hemodynamic monitoring plays a pivotal role in critical care settings, where understanding the cardiovascular status of patients can mean the difference between life and death. It provides real-time insights into a patient's circulatory health, offering a detailed view of how well the heart is functioning and whether the tissues are being adequately perfused with oxygen-rich blood. The primary aim of hemodynamic monitoring is to support clinical decision-making by enabling timely diagnosis, guiding therapeutic interventions, and assessing response to treatment.

Sepsis, heart failure, or shock can all quickly alter hemodynamic parameters in critically ill individuals. These changes may not always be obvious on a physical examination. That's where hemodynamic monitoring comes in handy, since it allows clinicians to identify tiny changes in blood pressure, cardiac output, and vascular resistance, allowing for exact treatment modifications. Let's look at some important responsibilities that hemodynamic monitoring plays in critical care:

1. Detecting Hemodynamic Instability Early

One of the most crucial roles of hemodynamic monitoring is the early detection of hemodynamic instability, which can precede significant clinical deterioration. Changes in cardiac output, central venous pressure (CVP), or mixed venous oxygen saturation (SvO2) can serve as early warning signs of conditions like:

- **Septic Shock:** Low cardiac output with high SVR.
- **Hypovolemic Shock:** Reduced preload and low stroke volume.
- **Cardiogenic Shock:** Increased preload and afterload due to poor cardiac contractility.

- Early detection helps clinicians intervene proactively, often before other clinical symptoms manifest, thereby improving patient outcomes.

2. Guiding Fluid and Vasopressor Therapy

Hemodynamic monitoring is fundamental in guiding fluid therapy and the administration of vasoactive medications. For example:

- **Fluid Resuscitation:** By monitoring parameters like CVP, pulmonary artery occlusion pressure (PAOP), and stroke volume variation (SVV), clinicians can determine if a patient is fluid-responsive and tailor fluid administration accordingly.
- **Vasopressor Therapy:** In patients with distributive or cardiogenic shock, hemodynamic data like systemic vascular resistance (SVR) and mean arterial pressure (MAP) guide the use of vasopressors such as norepinephrine or vasopressin.

This targeted approach ensures that patients receive appropriate treatment without the risks of fluid overload or inadequate perfusion.

3. Evaluating Cardiac Function and Contractility

Hemodynamic monitoring can provide detailed information about the heart's pumping ability and overall function. Parameters such as:

- **Cardiac Index (CI):** CO adjusted for body surface area.
- **Ejection Fraction (EF):** Percentage of blood ejected from the ventricles with each beat.
- **Stroke Volume Variation (SVV):** Changes in stroke volume during the respiratory cycle.
  These metrics are particularly useful in assessing myocardial contractility in patients with heart failure, myocardial infarction, or post-cardiac surgery. Based on this information, clinicians can adjust inotropes or vasodilators to improve heart function.

4. Assessing Oxygen Delivery and Tissue Perfusion

In critically ill patients, ensuring adequate tissue oxygenation is paramount. Hemodynamic monitoring allows for the assessment of key indicators of tissue perfusion and oxygenation, such as:

- **Mixed Venous Oxygen Saturation (SvO2):** Reflects the balance between oxygen delivery and consumption.
- **Lactate Levels:** Indicates tissue hypoperfusion if elevated.
- **Venous-to-Arterial CO2 Gap:** A marker of microcirculatory dysfunction.

- Monitoring these parameters enables early recognition of impaired oxygen delivery and prompts interventions to improve tissue perfusion, such as optimizing cardiac output or hemoglobin levels.

5. Optimizing Mechanical Ventilation and Weaning

In patients on mechanical ventilation, hemodynamic monitoring can be essential in assessing the cardiovascular impact of positive pressure ventilation. For instance, high levels of positive end-expiratory pressure (PEEP) can affect venous return and reduce cardiac output. By monitoring preload and stroke volume, clinicians can make informed adjustments to ventilation settings.

Moreover, hemodynamic monitoring can guide the weaning process by identifying hemodynamic stability or instability during spontaneous breathing trials (SBTs).

6. Managing Complex Critical Scenarios

Hemodynamic monitoring is indispensable in managing complex cases like:
- **Multisystem Organ Failure:** Identifying primary hemodynamic deficits and targeting therapy.
- **High-Risk Surgeries:** Perioperative monitoring in cardiac or major vascular surgeries to prevent intraoperative and postoperative complications.
- **Burn Patients:** Monitoring hemodynamic changes associated with massive fluid shifts.

7. Personalized Medicine: Tailoring Interventions to Patient Needs

Finally, one of the most valuable aspects of hemodynamic monitoring is the ability to implement personalized medicine. Every critically ill patient is unique, and standardized protocols may not always apply. By continuously tracking hemodynamic parameters, clinicians can tailor interventions — such as adjusting fluid, vasopressor, or inotrope therapy — to match the patient's current condition.

In summary, hemodynamic monitoring is a cornerstone of critical care practice, providing invaluable information about the cardiovascular status of critically ill patients. It enables clinicians to detect hemodynamic instability early, tailor fluid and medication therapies, evaluate cardiac function, and ensure adequate tissue perfusion. By mastering these concepts, healthcare professionals can significantly improve patient outcomes and ensure safe, effective critical care management.

CHAPTER TWO

Tools of the Trade

Hemodynamic monitoring is only as effective as the equipment used to measure, record, and interpret the various parameters. As technology has advanced, so has the sophistication of monitoring tools, ranging from simple non-invasive devices to complex invasive systems. Understanding these tools and how to use them correctly is essential for ensuring accurate measurements and, ultimately, safe patient care.

In this chapter, we'll take a deep dive into the various types of equipment commonly used for hemodynamic monitoring in critical care settings. We'll discuss the fundamental components, from basic blood pressure cuffs to more advanced technologies like arterial lines, pulmonary artery catheters, and continuous cardiac output monitors. It's crucial to have a solid grasp of each piece of equipment, its purpose, and how to set it up accurately to obtain reliable data.

Additionally, we'll cover practical considerations like equipment calibration, troubleshooting common problems, and maintaining sterility to minimize the risk of hospital-acquired infections. The proper use of monitoring equipment not only safeguards patient outcomes but also provides clinicians with a real-time window into the cardiovascular health of their patients.

whether or not you're a novice or an experienced healthcare professional, this chapter will provide you with the knowledge and confidence you need to use hemodynamic monitoring devices effectively. Let's begin by looking at the various tools of the trade and the key practices for ensuring their optimal use.

OVERVIEW OF MONITORING EQUIPMENT

Hemodynamic monitoring relies on a diverse array of equipment to provide a comprehensive picture of a patient's cardiovascular status. Each piece of equipment, from basic to advanced, serves a unique function, helping clinicians to accurately assess parameters like blood pressure, cardiac output, and oxygen saturation. The selection of monitoring equipment depends on the clinical scenario, the patient's condition, and the level of detail required for effective management.

This section will cover the various types of monitoring equipment used in critical care, categorized into **non-invasive**, **minimally invasive**, and **invasive** tools. Each type has its own advantages, limitations, and appropriate clinical indications. Understanding the strengths and applications of these tools is vital for making informed decisions about patient care.

1. Non-Invasive Monitoring Equipment

Non-invasive monitoring techniques are often the first step in assessing a patient's hemodynamic status. They are relatively simple to use, pose no risk of infection, and are ideal for continuous bedside monitoring. Common non-invasive equipment includes:

- **Blood Pressure Cuffs (Sphygmomanometers):**
    a. Measure arterial blood pressure (systolic, diastolic, and mean).
    b. Easy to use and widely available in different sizes.
- **Pulse Oximeters:**
    a. Measure oxygen saturation (SpO2) and provide a pulse rate.
    b. Useful for assessing oxygenation but not a direct indicator of cardiac output.
- **Doppler Ultrasound:**
    a. Utilizes sound waves to estimate blood flow and velocity.

b. Can be used for peripheral vascular assessments or echocardiography.
- **Non-Invasive Cardiac Output Monitoring**:
  a. Systems like bioimpedance or bioreactance provide cardiac output estimations.
  b. Suitable for patients where invasive monitoring is not warranted.

While non-invasive methods are safe and easy to use, they may not provide the level of detail required for managing critically ill patients. That's where more advanced, minimally invasive, and invasive tools come into play.

2. Minimally Invasive Monitoring Equipment

Minimally invasive methods offer more detailed information than non-invasive tools without the high risk of complications associated with invasive devices. These include:

- **Arterial Catheters (Art Lines)**:
  - Provide continuous, real-time arterial blood pressure measurements.
  - Allow for frequent arterial blood sampling for blood gas analysis.
  - Typically inserted into the radial or femoral artery.
- **Central Venous Catheters (CVCs)**:
  - Measure central venous pressure (CVP), which reflects right atrial pressure and overall fluid status.
  - Useful for administering medications and central venous blood sampling.
- **Esophageal Doppler Monitors**:
  - Measure blood flow and cardiac output using a probe placed in the esophagus.
  - Less invasive than pulmonary artery catheters and useful for perioperative monitoring.

These devices are more accurate than non-invasive tools and are particularly useful in unstable patients where subtle changes in hemodynamic status need to be closely monitored.

3. Invasive Monitoring Equipment

Invasive monitoring tools are the gold standard for critically ill patients requiring detailed hemodynamic assessment. They provide precise measurements of various parameters, but their use comes with higher risks, such as infection, bleeding, or vascular damage. Common invasive tools include:

1. **Pulmonary Artery Catheters (PACs):**
    a. Also known as Swan-Ganz catheters, they measure pulmonary artery pressure, cardiac output, and pulmonary capillary wedge pressure (PCWP).
    b. Ideal for managing complex cases like cardiogenic shock or severe heart failure.
2. **Transpulmonary Thermodilution Devices:**
    a. Measure cardiac output using temperature changes after injecting a cold saline bolus.
    b. Useful for measuring extravascular lung water and systemic vascular resistance.
3. **Intra-aortic Balloon Pumps (IABP):**
    a. Provide mechanical support for patients with severe left ventricular failure.
    b. Improve coronary perfusion and decrease afterload by inflating and deflating a balloon within the aorta.
4. **Left Ventricular Assist Devices (LVADs):**
    a. Used in patients with end-stage heart failure to maintain cardiac output.
    b. Require comprehensive monitoring and skilled management.

The choice of invasive monitoring device depends on the clinical condition, the need for detailed hemodynamic data, and the risk-benefit ratio for the patient.

Choosing the Right Equipment: Considerations for Clinicians

Selecting the right monitoring tool involves balancing accuracy, safety, and clinical need. Factors to consider include:

- **Patient's Condition:** Is the patient hemodynamically stable or unstable?
- **Level of Detail Required:** Do you need detailed cardiac output measurements or basic blood pressure monitoring?
- **Risk of Complications:** Is the patient at high risk for infection, bleeding, or vascular injury?
- **Ease of Use and Availability:** Are the resources and trained

personnel available to use and maintain the equipment?

By understanding the capabilities and limitations of each type of monitoring device, healthcare professionals can select the most appropriate tool for each patient, ensuring optimal outcomes.

Monitoring Equipment	Category	Pros	Cons	Clinical Applications
Pulse Oximeter	Non-Invasive	Easy to use, provides quick oxygen saturation readings	Can be inaccurate in cases of poor circulation or movement	Monitoring oxygen levels in patients with respiratory issues
ECG (Electrocardiogram)	Non-Invasive	Non-invasive heart rhythm monitoring	Limited to electrical activity, doesn't assess blood flow	Detecting arrhythmias, ischemia, and monitoring cardiac health
NIBP (Non-Invasive Blood Pressure)	Non-Invasive	Simple and safe for routine blood pressure measurement	May not be as accurate during motion or in critical patients	Routine blood pressure monitoring
Continuous Glucose Monitor (CGM)	Minimally Invasive	Provides real-time blood glucose data	Requires sensor insertion, potential for irritation	Managing diabetes, monitoring glucose trends in critical care
Arterial Line	Invasive	Continuous and accurate blood pressure monitoring	Risk of infection, requires skilled placement	Used in critical care for hemodynamic monitoring
Central Venous Catheter (CVC)	Invasive	Measures central venous pressure, used for medication delivery	Risk of infection, pneumothorax, and thrombosis	Fluid management, delivery of vasoactive agents, central access
Pulmonary Artery Catheter	Invasive	Comprehensive hemodynamic data, assesses cardiac output	High risk of complications, requires experienced personnel	Hemodynamic monitoring in critically ill patients
EEG (Electroencephalogram)	Non-Invasive	Assesses electrical brain activity	Can be prone to artifact and interference	Monitoring for seizures, assessing brain activity in coma patients
ICP Monitor (Intracranial Pressure)	Invasive	Direct measurement of intracranial pressure	High risk of infection and bleeding	Monitoring in traumatic brain injury, assessing cerebral perfusion
Fetal Heart Rate Monitor	Non-Invasive/ Minimally Invasive	Provides information on fetal wellbeing	Can cause discomfort, limitations in maternal obesity	Monitoring fetal health during labor

Table 1: Monitoring Equipment Details

SETTING UP AND CALIBRATING EQUIPMENT SAFELY

Proper setup and calibration of hemodynamic monitoring equipment are critical steps that ensure the accuracy and reliability of the data collected. Incorrect calibration or poor setup can lead to erroneous readings, misinterpretation, and ultimately, inappropriate clinical decisions. For healthcare professionals, mastering the setup and calibration of monitoring devices is an essential skill that requires attention to detail and adherence to best practices.

In this section, we'll break down the step-by-step procedures for setting up commonly used hemodynamic monitoring devices. We'll also cover the principles of zeroing and leveling, which are vital for maintaining accurate pressure measurements. These procedures are foundational in reducing measurement errors and ensuring patient safety.

GENERAL PRINCIPLES OF EQUIPMENT SETUP

Before setting up any hemodynamic monitoring device, follow these general guidelines:

1. **Ensure Proper Sterility and Hygiene**:
   - Always practice sterile techniques to minimize the risk of infection.
   - Use appropriate protective equipment, such as sterile gloves, gowns, and face shields.
2. **Verify Equipment Functionality**:
   - Check for any signs of wear or damage in cables, connectors, or sensors.
   - Test the device's power supply and battery status.
3. **Have the Right Equipment Ready**:
   - Gather all necessary supplies, including pressure transducers, IV fluids, catheter kits, and syringes.
   - Familiarize yourself with the device's manual and operational guidelines.

Equipment Type Step	1: Initial Setup Step	2: Sensor Check Step	3: Calibration Adjustment	Step 4: Data Verification	Step 5: Final Confirmation	Completed (✓)
Blood Pressure Monitor	Attach cuff to patient's upper arm	Verify cuff inflation and deflation	Adjust zero reference point if needed	Check readings against known value	Confirm stability and accuracy	
Pulse Oximeter	Place sensor on patient's finger	Ensure correct placement and light path	Calibrate sensor sensitivity	Compare with manual pulse count	Verify SpO2 value is within expected range	
ECG Monitor	Connect electrodes to the chest	Test electrode contact quality	Adjust baseline if drift is observed	Check against simulated waveform	Ensure consistent signal capture	
Thermometer	Place probe in designated area	Confirm probe is intact	Set calibration offset	Measure against a known standard	Confirm temperature stability	
Capnography Device	Connect to airway circuit	Validate sensor responsiveness	Calibrate CO_2 levels using standard gas	Review waveform for anomalies	Confirm end-tidal CO_2 is accurate	

Table 2.0: Calibration Checklist

1. Setting Up an Arterial Line (Art Line)

Arterial lines are commonly used for continuous blood pressure monitoring and arterial blood gas sampling. Here's a step-by-step guide for setting up an Art Line:

1. **Prepare the Pressure Transducer System:**
   - Attach the pressure tubing to a pressurized bag of normal saline (300 mmHg).
   - Connect the tubing to the transducer and ensure there are no air bubbles in the line.
2. **Position the Transducer at the Correct Level:**
   - Level the transducer to the phlebostatic axis (approximately the 4th intercostal space, mid-axillary line) to align it with the right atrium.
   - Secure the transducer at this level to avoid shifts that can cause inaccurate readings.
3. **Zero the Transducer:**
   - Open the transducer's stopcock to air (atmospheric pressure) and press the zero button on the monitor.
   - Verify that the display reads zero before connecting to the patient.
4. **Insert the Arterial Catheter:**
   - Use sterile technique to insert the catheter into the radial or femoral artery.
   - Confirm arterial waveform on the monitor once connected.
5. **Check for Accurate Waveforms:**
   - Ensure that the waveform has a distinct dicrotic notch, indicating proper placement.
   - Monitor for complications such as damping, which could indicate kinking or obstruction.

2. Setting Up a Central Venous Catheter (CVC)

CVCs are used to measure central venous pressure (CVP) and for administering medications. The setup process is similar to arterial lines but requires extra caution due to the risk of complications like pneumothorax. Steps include:

1. **Flush and Prime the Pressure Tubing System**:
   - Attach the transducer tubing to a pressurized saline bag and prime the system.
   - Eliminate air bubbles from the tubing.
2. **Position the Patient**:
   - Place the patient in the Trendelenburg position (head down) to facilitate catheter insertion and reduce the risk of air embolism.
3. **Zero and Calibrate the Transducer**:
   - Level the transducer at the phlebostatic axis, similar to the arterial line setup.
   - Zero the transducer to ensure accurate CVP readings.
4. **Insert the CVC Under Ultrasound Guidance**:
   - Use sterile technique and ultrasound guidance to insert the CVC into the internal jugular or subclavian vein.
   - Secure the catheter and connect it to the transducer system.
5. **Obtain a Baseline CVP Measurement**:
   - Confirm correct placement by visualizing the waveform and obtaining a baseline CVP measurement (typically 2-6 mmHg).

3. Setting Up Pulmonary Artery Catheters (PACs)

Pulmonary artery catheters (Swan-Ganz catheters) are advanced monitoring devices used for detailed hemodynamic assessment. Setting up a PAC involves:

1. **Assemble the Pressure Monitoring System**:
   - Prime the PAC with sterile saline and connect to a pressure transducer system.
2. **Position and Zero the Transducer**:
   - As with other devices, level the transducer at the

phlebostatic axis and zero it to atmospheric pressure.
3. **Insert the PAC Through a Central Line**:
- Insert the PAC through a pre-established CVC in the jugular or subclavian vein.
- Monitor the waveform as the catheter is advanced through the right atrium, right ventricle, and into the pulmonary artery.
4. **Inflate the Balloon**:
- Inflate the balloon at the catheter tip to "float" it into the pulmonary artery.
- Confirm placement by observing a distinct pulmonary artery waveform.
5. **Measure Key Hemodynamic Parameters**:
- Use the PAC to obtain readings for pulmonary artery pressure (PAP), pulmonary capillary wedge pressure (PCWP), and cardiac output.

4. Setting Up Non-Invasive Devices (Blood Pressure Cuffs, Pulse Oximeters)

While non-invasive devices are simpler to set up, they still require proper placement and calibration:

1. **Place the Device Correctly**:
- For blood pressure cuffs, ensure the cuff size is appropriate and positioned at heart level.
- For pulse oximeters, ensure a snug fit on the finger or ear without excessive movement.
2. **Calibrate for Baseline Readings**:
- Some devices allow for baseline calibration; follow the manufacturer's instructions.
3. **Monitor for Accuracy**:
- Regularly assess for conditions that may interfere with readings, such as poor perfusion, cold extremities, or motion artifacts.

TROUBLESHOOTING TIPS FOR COMMON ISSUES

- **Zero Drift**: Re-zero the transducer system if readings are inconsistent.
- **Waveform Abnormalities**: Check for kinks, air bubbles, or incorrect transducer positioning.
- **Infection Control**: Follow strict aseptic techniques and change dressings regularly to minimize infection risks.

Troubleshooting Common Equipment Issues

Even the most advanced hemodynamic monitoring equipment can encounter problems that affect the quality and reliability of the data. Being able to troubleshoot these issues effectively is a crucial skill for healthcare professionals. This section will cover common equipment issues, potential causes, and step-by-step solutions to restore accurate functionality.

1. Zeroing and Calibration Issues

One of the most frequent problems encountered is inaccurate zeroing or calibration of pressure transducers, which can lead to erroneous readings. This can result from incorrect leveling, transducer drift, or environmental factors.

- **Problem**: The waveform appears flat or distorted, or the values do not match clinical expectations.
- **Potential Causes**:
    - Incorrect transducer leveling.
    - Air bubbles in the system.
    - Inadequate zeroing of the transducer.

- **Solution**:
  - Recheck the level of the transducer at the phlebostatic axis.
  - Remove any air bubbles by gently tapping the tubing and using the stopcock to flush.
  - Re-zero the transducer by opening it to atmospheric pressure and verifying the monitor reads zero.

2. Waveform Dampening or Exaggeration

Dampening or exaggeration of waveforms is a common issue that can occur with both arterial and central venous pressure monitoring systems.

- **Problem**: The waveform is either smoothed out (dampened) or has exaggerated peaks (overdamped).
- **Potential Causes**:
  - Air bubbles or blood clots in the tubing.
  - Kinked or overly compliant tubing.
  - Poor catheter placement or vessel spasm.
- **Solution**:
  - Inspect the tubing for kinks, clots, or bubbles and remove any obstructions.
  - Replace any tubing that appears excessively soft or compliant.
  - Reposition the catheter if necessary, ensuring it is correctly placed.

3. Artifact Interference

Artifacts are abnormal signals on the monitor that do not represent true physiological events and can mislead clinical interpretation.

- **Problem**: Erratic or spiking readings that do not correspond with the patient's clinical status.
- **Potential Causes**:
  - Patient movement or shivering.

- Electrical interference from nearby devices.
- Loose connections in the monitoring system.
- **Solution**:
  - Minimize patient movement if possible and ensure the patient is comfortable.
  - Check for loose connections or damaged cables and replace if needed.
  - Relocate equipment if there's suspected electrical interference.

4. Catheter Occlusion or Malfunction

If the catheter is occluded or malfunctions, it can prevent accurate pressure transmission and may pose a risk to the patient.

- **Problem**: Sudden loss of waveform or pressure readings.
- **Potential Causes**:
  - Catheter kinking or displacement.
  - Thrombus formation at the catheter tip.
  - Clogged line or closed stopcock.
- **Solution**:
  - Assess for kinks and gently adjust the catheter if needed.
  - Use heparinized saline to flush the line if clotting is suspected (following institutional protocol).
  - Reposition or replace the catheter if it is dislodged or malfunctioning.

5. Equipment Malfunction

Sometimes, the issue lies within the equipment itself rather than the setup or patient factors.

- **Problem**: The monitor is unresponsive or displays erroneous values despite correct setup.
- **Potential Causes**:
  - Software glitches or outdated firmware.

- Battery or power supply failure.
- Defective transducers or cables.
- **Solution**:
  - Restart the monitor and verify that all software and firmware are up-to-date.
  - Replace the power source or use an alternative power supply.
  - Test with a new transducer or cables to isolate the faulty component.

6. Infection Control Concerns

Even with a perfect equipment setup, the risk of infection can increase due to the contamination of monitoring lines.

- **Problem**: Increased incidence of line-associated infections or sepsis.
- **Potential Causes**:
  - Breaches in sterility during line insertion.
  - Infrequent dressing changes or line maintenance.
  - Contaminated equipment or fluids.
- **Solution**:
  - Follow strict aseptic techniques during insertion and line handling.
  - Change dressings and flush lines according to hospital protocols.
  - Use sterile fluids and replace contaminated components promptly.

MAINTAINING STERILITY AND MINIMIZING INFECTIONS

One of the most critical aspects of using hemodynamic monitoring equipment is ensuring that sterility is maintained throughout the setup and monitoring process. Given that these systems involve direct access to the patient's vascular system, any breach in sterility can introduce harmful pathogens, leading to potentially life-threatening infections such as catheter-associated bloodstream infections (CLABSIs) or sepsis.

In this section, we'll look at recommended practices for keeping the environment sterile, reducing infection risks, and handling hemodynamic monitoring equipment and catheters securely.

1. Aseptic Technique: The Foundation of Sterility

Aseptic technique involves all the measures taken to prevent contamination from pathogens, ensuring that everything that comes in contact with the patient is sterile. This starts from the moment of catheter insertion and extends throughout the duration of monitoring.

- **Key Steps for Aseptic Technique**:
  → **Hand Hygiene**: Always perform thorough handwashing with antiseptic soap or use alcohol-based hand sanitizer before any procedure.
  → **Sterile Gloves and Gown**: Wear sterile gloves and, when indicated, a sterile gown when inserting or handling invasive lines.
  → **Sterile Draping**: Use sterile drapes to create a

barrier between the catheter site and the surrounding environment.

→ **Disinfection of Skin**: Use a chlorhexidine-based solution to cleanse the insertion site. Allow it to dry completely before proceeding.

2. Best Practices for Catheter Insertion

The insertion of a catheter is a delicate procedure that requires meticulous attention to sterility. Following a standardized protocol can help reduce the risk of contamination.

- **Site Selection**: Prefer peripheral sites or the subclavian vein for central lines, as they are associated with a lower risk of infection compared to the femoral site.
- **Insertion Kit**: Use a pre-packaged sterile insertion kit to minimize the need for additional handling of individual sterile components.
- **Sterile Field**: Ensure that all instruments, catheters, and equipment are placed within a sterile field. Any breach in sterility (e.g., a non-sterile object touching a sterile component) should prompt immediate replacement of the contaminated item.

3. Post-Insertion Care and Line Maintenance

Maintaining a sterile environment following successful catheter insertion is critical to infection prevention. Regular maintenance and attentive care for the catheter and its connections can greatly minimize infection rates.

- **Dressing Changes**: Change catheter dressings at regular intervals (typically every 7 days for transparent dressings and every 48 hours for gauze dressings) or sooner if they become damp, soiled, or loosened.
  → **Sterile Technique for Dressing Changes**: Use aseptic technique when changing dressings. Disinfect

the catheter site with chlorhexidine and allow it to dry before applying a new dressing.
- **Line Flushing**: Regularly flush the catheter line with sterile, heparinized saline (as per hospital protocol) to maintain patency and minimize the risk of clot formation. Use single-use vials or pre-filled syringes to avoid contamination.
- **Catheter Hub Care**: Disinfect catheter hubs and needleless connectors with alcohol or chlorhexidine before each access. Avoid frequent manipulation of these components to reduce the risk of contamination.

4. Handling and Replacing Equipment

Equipment used in hemodynamic monitoring, such as pressure transducers, flush systems, and tubing, should be handled with care to prevent contamination. Any component that is compromised should be replaced immediately.

- **Sterile Handling of Transducers**: Always use sterile gloves when attaching or detaching pressure transducers. Replace the transducer set according to institutional guidelines, typically every 96 hours.
- **Avoid Reuse of Single-Use Equipment**: Never reuse single-use items such as syringes, tubing, or flush bags. Reuse increases the risk of introducing pathogens into the system.
- **Minimizing Line Manipulation**: Limit unnecessary line manipulation or disconnection, as each access increases the risk of contamination. Use closed systems whenever possible to reduce exposure.

5. Recognizing and Managing Infection Risks

Even with rigorous adherence to sterile technique, the risk of infection is never zero. Early recognition of infection signs and prompt intervention are crucial to preventing severe complications.

- **Signs of Infection**:
  - Redness, swelling, or tenderness at the catheter insertion site.
  - Purulent drainage from the site.
  - Sudden onset of fever, chills, or hypotension in the absence of other infection sources.
- **Actions to Take**:
  - Immediately notify the healthcare provider if infection is suspected.
  - Discontinue the use of the suspected catheter and send the tip for culture, if indicated.
  - Initiate empirical antibiotic therapy as per hospital protocol until the specific pathogen is identified.

6. Strategies for Reducing Catheter-Associated Infections

Healthcare facilities can adopt additional strategies to further reduce the risk of catheter-associated infections. These include the use of antimicrobial-impregnated catheters, chlorhexidine-impregnated dressings, and dedicated catheter insertion and maintenance teams.

- **Antimicrobial Catheters**: Consider using antimicrobial or antiseptic-impregnated catheters for patients requiring prolonged catheterization or for those at high risk of infection.
- **Catheter Care Bundles**: Implementing standardized catheter care bundles, which include a set of evidence-based practices, has been shown to significantly reduce infection rates.

CHAPTER THREE

Core Hemodynamic Parameters Explained

Hemodynamic monitoring relies on a set of core parameters that reflect the functionality and status of a patient's cardiovascular system. These parameters provide critical insights into the patient's fluid balance, cardiac performance, and vascular resistance, all of which are essential for guiding clinical decision-making. Understanding these key metrics enables clinicians to make informed choices regarding fluid therapy, medication administration, and other interventions to optimize patient outcomes.

This chapter will provide an in-depth explanation of the most commonly used hemodynamic parameters, including Central Venous Pressure (CVP), Mean Arterial Pressure (MAP), Cardiac Output (CO) and Cardiac Index (CI), Pulmonary Capillary Wedge Pressure (PCWP), and Systemic and Pulmonary Vascular Resistance (SVR and PVR). Each section will cover what these parameters represent, how they are measured, their normal ranges, and what deviations from these norms may indicate about a patient's cardiovascular health.

By the end of this chapter, you will have a solid understanding of the fundamental hemodynamic measurements and their clinical implications, making it easier to analyze complex monitoring data and apply it to real-time patient management.

CENTRAL VENOUS PRESSURE (CVP)

Central Venous Pressure (CVP) is one of the fundamental hemodynamic parameters used to evaluate the status of a patient's fluid volume and right ventricular function. It measures the pressure within the thoracic vena cava or right atrium, providing insights into the amount of blood returning to the heart (preload) and the heart's ability to pump this blood into the pulmonary circulation. Essentially, CVP serves as an indicator of the balance between the volume of blood returning to the heart and the capacity of the right ventricle to accommodate and eject this blood.

1. Understanding CVP: What Does It Measure?

CVP reflects the pressure exerted by the venous blood in the large veins leading to the heart, specifically the superior vena cava (SVC) and right atrium. It is expressed in millimeters of mercury (mmHg) and typically measured through a central venous catheter inserted into one of the major veins (e.g., internal jugular or subclavian vein).

Normal Range:

- A normal CVP value ranges from **2 to 8 mmHg**.

Low CVP Values:

- A CVP value below 2 mmHg may suggest hypovolemia (e.g., dehydration or significant blood loss) or venodilation, which may require fluid resuscitation.

High CVP Values:

- A CVP value above 8 mmHg can indicate fluid overload, right ventricular failure, or increased intrathoracic pressure, which may necessitate diuresis or other interventions.

2. Why Is CVP Important?

CVP is an essential component in assessing a patient's fluid status, making it a valuable tool in critical care settings. It helps clinicians determine whether a patient needs more fluids, has an adequate preload, or is suffering from conditions such as heart failure or shock. However, it's important to note that CVP should never be used in isolation. It should be considered alongside other parameters, clinical assessments, and patient-specific factors.

Clinical Uses of CVP:

- **Fluid Management**: Guides fluid therapy decisions in patients with suspected hypovolemia or fluid overload.
- **Assessment of Right Ventricular Function**: Helps evaluate the right side of the heart, especially in cases of right-sided heart failure or pulmonary hypertension.
- **Monitoring During Surgery or Critical Illness**: Provides real-time information on the patient's hemodynamic status in complex surgical procedures and critical care settings.

3. How is CVP Measured?

CVP is measured using a central venous catheter (also called a central line) connected to a transducer system. The catheter is inserted through a large vein (commonly the internal jugular or subclavian vein) and advanced until the tip is positioned in the lower part of the superior vena cava, near the right atrium.

Key Steps in Measuring CVP:

1. **Insertion of Central Venous Catheter**: Performed

under sterile conditions using ultrasound guidance to avoid complications.
2. **Zeroing the Transducer**: The transducer is calibrated at the level of the patient's phlebostatic axis (typically the 4th intercostal space at the mid-axillary line) to ensure accurate readings.
3. **Reading the CVP Value**: The pressure waveform is displayed on a monitor, and the mean value is noted.

4. Interpretation and Clinical Application of CVP Values

Understanding the nuances of CVP values is crucial for appropriate clinical decision-making. It is important to integrate CVP data with clinical assessments and other hemodynamic measurements to get a comprehensive view of the patient's condition.

- **Low CVP (Below 2 mmHg)**: Often suggests decreased venous return, hypovolemia, or vasodilation. Common causes include dehydration, hemorrhage, or septic shock.
- **Normal CVP (2–8 mmHg)**: Indicates a balanced fluid status and right ventricular function under normal physiological conditions.
- **High CVP (Above 8 mmHg)**: Can indicate conditions such as right heart failure, pulmonary hypertension, fluid overload, or obstructive pathologies like tension pneumothorax or cardiac tamponade.

Management Based on CVP:

- **Low CVP**: Consider fluid administration to restore intravascular volume.
- **High CVP**: Investigate for signs of right ventricular dysfunction, fluid overload, or increased thoracic pressure. Management may include diuretics, positive inotropes, or addressing the underlying cause (e.g., pericardiocentesis for tamponade).

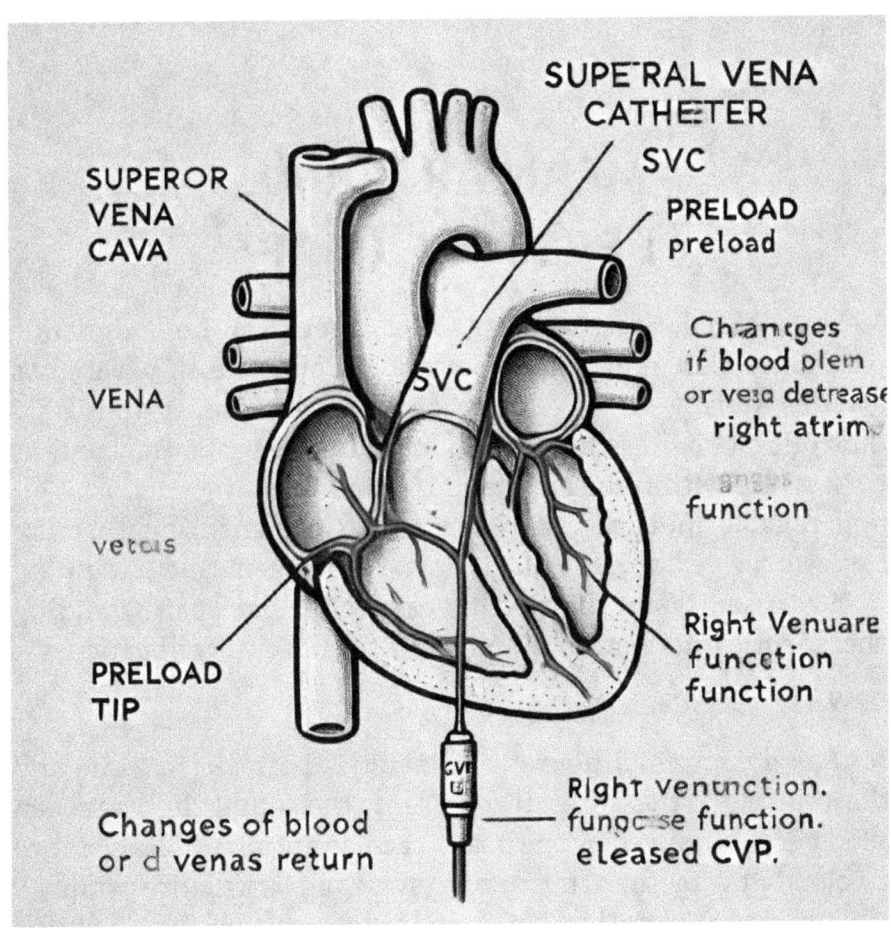

Figure 3.1: Central Venous Catheter Placement for Measuring CVP

MEAN ARTERIAL PRESSURE (MAP)

Mean Arterial Pressure (MAP) is a critical hemodynamic parameter that represents the average pressure in a patient's arteries during a single cardiac cycle. Unlike systolic and diastolic blood pressures, which measure the peaks and troughs of pressure within the arteries, MAP provides a more consistent and reliable indicator of tissue perfusion, ensuring that the organs receive adequate blood flow and oxygen. Understanding MAP is essential for monitoring cardiovascular health, guiding therapeutic interventions, and managing critically ill patients.

1. What is MAP?

MAP is a computed figure that includes both the systolic and diastolic blood pressures. It represents the equilibrium between blood flow produced by the heart (cardiac output) and resistance to blood flow by the artery walls (systemic vascular resistance). This measure is critical for sustaining organ perfusion and is commonly used to assess the efficacy of circulatory support.

The formula for MAP Calculation:

MAP is generally calculated using the following formula:

$$MAP = \text{Diastolic BP} + \frac{(\text{Systolic BP} - \text{Diastolic BP})}{3}$$

Where:

- **Systolic BP** = Systolic Blood Pressure
- **Diastolic BP** = Diastolic Blood Pressure

2. What is the Normal Range for MAP?

The normal range for MAP is typically between **70 and 100 mmHg**. This range ensures adequate perfusion of vital organs such as the brain, kidneys, and heart. Maintaining a MAP above 60 mmHg is generally considered necessary to prevent organ ischemia and ensure cellular oxygenation.

- **Low MAP (< 60 mmHg)**: Indicates poor perfusion pressure, which may lead to organ hypoperfusion, particularly in the brain and kidneys.
- **High MAP (> 100 mmHg)**: Suggests increased systemic resistance or elevated cardiac output, potentially resulting in damage to arterial walls over time.

3. Why is MAP Important?

MAP is more than just an average blood pressure; it is a vital measure of the driving force that propels blood through the circulatory system and into the organs. For this reason, MAP is a primary parameter used in critical care to guide treatment decisions, particularly in cases of shock, sepsis, or traumatic injury.

Clinical Uses of MAP:

- **Guiding Vasopressor Therapy**: In critically ill patients, maintaining an optimal MAP is essential to ensure adequate perfusion, especially during shock or hypotensive states.
- **Assessing Organ Perfusion**: MAP is a direct indicator of perfusion pressure, making it a key metric for ensuring that organs like the kidneys and brain receive sufficient blood flow.
- **Monitoring During Surgery**: Intraoperative monitoring of MAP helps avoid periods of hypoperfusion or hypertension, reducing the risk of complications.

4. How is MAP Measured?

MAP can be measured directly using invasive arterial lines

or estimated non-invasively using oscillometric blood pressure monitors. In critical care settings, invasive methods are preferred due to their accuracy and ability to provide continuous readings.

Measurement Methods:

- **Invasive Method**: An arterial catheter (usually placed in the radial or femoral artery) is connected to a transducer that provides real-time blood pressure waveforms. This method is highly accurate and used in intensive care and surgical settings.
- **Non-Invasive Method**: Calculated indirectly using a standard blood pressure cuff. Although less precise, this method is widely used in general practice and for less critically ill patients.

5. Interpretation of MAP in Clinical Scenarios

MAP is a valuable indicator for diagnosing and managing a variety of cardiovascular conditions. Its interpretation should always be integrated with the overall clinical picture, including patient history, physical examination, and other hemodynamic parameters.

- **Low MAP**: Can result from hypovolemia, cardiac failure, or severe sepsis, indicating that perfusion to vital organs is inadequate. The treatment goal is often to restore intravascular volume or improve cardiac output using fluids, inotropes, or vasopressors.
- **High MAP**: May be caused by excessive vasoconstriction, elevated cardiac output, or conditions such as hypertension. Management focuses on reducing systemic vascular resistance and addressing the underlying cause.

6. Clinical Applications of MAP in Different Conditions

- **Septic Shock**: Maintaining a MAP ≥ 65 mmHg is a critical target in the management of septic shock to ensure

adequate tissue perfusion.
- **Traumatic Brain Injury**: A MAP of 70–90 mmHg is typically recommended to optimize cerebral perfusion and prevent secondary brain injury.
- **Acute Kidney Injury**: Low MAP is associated with reduced renal perfusion, potentially leading to acute kidney injury. Maintaining an adequate MAP can help protect kidney function.

CARDIAC OUTPUT (CO) AND CARDIAC INDEX (CI)

Cardiac Output (CO) and Cardiac Index (CI) are two of the most fundamental hemodynamic parameters used to evaluate heart performance and the adequacy of blood circulation throughout the body. CO measures the total volume of blood pumped by the heart per minute, while CI adjusts that measurement based on the patient's body surface area, providing a more personalized assessment of cardiac function.

1. What is Cardiac Output (CO)?

Cardiac Output (CO) is the amount of blood that the heart pumps through the circulatory system in one minute. It is a critical determinant of how well oxygen and nutrients are delivered to the tissues and is a primary measure of cardiac performance. CO is a product of two key factors: heart rate (HR) and stroke volume (SV).

$$CO = HR \times SV$$

Where:

- **HR (Heart Rate)** = Number of heartbeats per minute
- **SV (Stroke Volume)** = Amount of blood pumped out of the heart with each beat

For example, if a patient's heart rate is 70 beats per minute and their stroke volume is 70 mL, the cardiac output would be:

$$CO = 70\,bpm \times 70\,mL = 4,900\,mL/min\ or\ 4.9\,L/min$$

2. Normal Ranges for Cardiac Output

A normal cardiac output for a healthy adult is approximately **4**

to 8 liters per minute. CO can vary significantly based on factors such as age, physical fitness, metabolic demands, and illness.

- **Low CO (< 4 L/min)**: Indicates impaired heart function or insufficient blood flow to meet the body's needs, often due to heart failure or shock.
- **High CO (> 8 L/min)**: Can result from conditions like sepsis, hyperthyroidism, or exercise, where the body requires more oxygen and nutrients.

3. What is Cardiac Index (CI)?

The Cardiac Index (CI) is an important refinement of cardiac output because it adjusts for the patient's body surface area (BSA), providing a more individualized evaluation of heart performance. By considering body size, the CI allows clinicians to compare cardiac performance across patients of varying sizes.

CI=CO/BSA

Where:

- **CO** = Cardiac Output
- **BSA** = Body Surface Area (in square meters)

Normal Range of CI: 2.5 to 4.0 L/min/m^2
If a patient's CI falls below 2.5 L/min/m^2, it may indicate poor cardiac performance, while values above 4.0 L/min/m^2 suggest increased cardiac activity.

4. Why Are CO and CI Important?

Both CO and CI are used to assess the heart's ability to supply the body with adequate blood flow. These parameters are particularly useful in critically ill patients, where even small changes can signify shifts in their cardiovascular status.

- **Low CO/CI**: May indicate heart failure, cardiogenic shock, or hypovolemia. Treatment often involves measures to improve cardiac contractility or increase circulating blood volume.

- **High CO/CI**: Can occur in conditions like sepsis or hypermetabolic states, and interventions focus on reducing heart stress and addressing the underlying cause.

5. How Are CO and CI Measured?

Several methods can be used to measure cardiac output, ranging from invasive to non-invasive techniques. In critical care, invasive methods like thermodilution and arterial pulse contour analysis provide real-time and accurate assessments, while less invasive methods are preferred in less acute settings.

Measurement Methods:

- **Thermodilution**: A catheter (often a pulmonary artery catheter) is inserted into the heart, and a cold saline solution is injected. The change in temperature as the blood mixes is measured, and cardiac output is calculated based on the rate of temperature change.
- **Pulse Contour Analysis**: An arterial line is used to continuously analyze the arterial pressure waveform, providing a real-time estimate of CO.
- **Non-invasive Techniques**: Methods like Doppler ultrasound or bioimpedance can estimate CO without inserting catheters into the heart, making them safer for routine monitoring.

6. Clinical Applications of CO and CI

Cardiac output and cardiac index are crucial for managing patients with various cardiovascular conditions, especially those in critical care settings where constant monitoring of heart function is needed.

- **Heart Failure**: Reduced CO or CI is a hallmark of heart failure, and therapies aim to improve cardiac contractility or reduce the heart's workload.
- **Shock**: In patients with septic, cardiogenic, or hypovolemic shock, maintaining an optimal CO/CI is essential for

ensuring adequate tissue perfusion and organ function.
- **Post-Operative Care**: After cardiac surgery, monitoring CO and CI can help detect complications such as low cardiac output syndrome, which can lead to poor organ perfusion and ischemia.
- **Sepsis**: In sepsis, CO often increases initially as the body tries to compensate for widespread vasodilation, but it may decrease as the condition progresses, necessitating fluid resuscitation and vasopressors.

PULMONARY CAPILLARY WEDGE PRESSURE (PCWP)

Pulmonary Capillary Wedge Pressure (PCWP), also referred to as the pulmonary artery wedge pressure (PAWP), is a crucial hemodynamic parameter that reflects left atrial pressure and is used to assess left ventricular function, especially in patients with heart failure. It is measured using a pulmonary artery (Swan-Ganz) catheter and offers valuable insights into the pressures and fluid status of the left side of the heart.

1. What is PCWP?

PCWP is an indirect measurement of the pressure in the left atrium and, by extension, the left ventricle's end-diastolic pressure (LVEDP). When a catheter is inserted into the pulmonary artery and its balloon tip is inflated, the blood flow is momentarily occluded, and the pressure transmitted from the left side of the heart can be recorded.

PCWP≈Left Atrial Pressure≈LVEDP

PCWP provides a reflection of how well the left side of the heart is functioning in terms of filling pressures and fluid balance. It helps clinicians assess fluid overload, left ventricular dysfunction, and the presence of pulmonary congestion.

2. Normal Range for PCWP

The normal PCWP for a healthy individual ranges between **6 to 12 mmHg**.

- **Low PCWP (< 6 mmHg)**: Indicates hypovolemia or inadequate filling pressures, which may occur in conditions such as dehydration, hemorrhage, or excessive

diuresis.
- **High PCWP (> 12 mmHg)**: Suggests elevated left atrial pressure, often associated with heart failure, mitral valve disease, or fluid overload.

3. Clinical Significance of PCWP

PCWP is a key diagnostic tool in managing patients with cardiovascular and respiratory diseases. It provides important information about:

- **Left Ventricular Function**: Elevated PCWP is a hallmark of left-sided heart failure, where the heart struggles to pump blood effectively, leading to a backup of pressure in the pulmonary circulation.
- **Fluid Status**: PCWP is often used to assess whether a patient is fluid overloaded or dehydrated, especially in critical care or heart failure management.
- **Pulmonary Congestion**: Elevated PCWP can result in pulmonary edema, a condition where fluid leaks into the lungs, causing difficulty breathing and impaired gas exchange.

4. How is PCWP Measured?

PCWP is measured using a pulmonary artery catheter (Swan-Ganz catheter), which is inserted through a central vein (often the internal jugular or subclavian vein) and advanced into the pulmonary artery. Once the catheter is in place, the balloon at the tip is inflated to occlude the blood flow, allowing pressure readings that reflect left atrial pressure.

Steps in Measuring PCWP:

- Insert the catheter into the pulmonary artery.
- Inflate the balloon at the catheter tip to "wedge" the vessel, temporarily occluding the blood flow.
- Record the pressure transmitted from the left atrium during the occlusion.

- Deflate the balloon and restore blood flow.

This measurement is invasive, and complications such as infection, pulmonary artery rupture, or arrhythmias can occur, so it is typically reserved for critically ill patients.

5. Clinical Applications of PCWP

PCWP is commonly used in several clinical scenarios, particularly in intensive care and cardiology settings, to guide treatment decisions and monitor disease progression.

- **Heart Failure**: Elevated PCWP is a key indicator of congestive heart failure (CHF), where the heart's inability to pump effectively leads to increased pressures and fluid accumulation in the lungs. In these patients, treatment focuses on reducing preload, often with diuretics and vasodilators, to lower PCWP and improve symptoms.
- **Acute Pulmonary Edema**: In patients with acute decompensated heart failure or severe mitral stenosis, PCWP can rise to dangerously high levels, causing fluid to leak into the lungs and impair gas exchange. Rapid interventions to reduce PCWP can be life-saving.
- **Shock States**: PCWP helps differentiate between different types of shock. In **cardiogenic shock**, PCWP is elevated due to poor cardiac output, while in **hypovolemic shock**, PCWP is low due to inadequate circulating volume.
- **Guiding Fluid Management**: In critically ill patients, managing fluid status is crucial. PCWP helps guide fluid resuscitation or diuresis to optimize cardiac function without causing pulmonary congestion.

6. Limitations of PCWP

While PCWP is a valuable parameter, it has limitations:

- It is an **invasive** procedure, carrying risks such as infection, catheter-related complications, or even pulmonary artery rupture.

- PCWP may be influenced by lung disease, positive pressure ventilation, or mitral valve dysfunction, making interpretation difficult in certain contexts.

As non-invasive alternatives continue to improve, the routine use of Swan-Ganz catheters for measuring PCWP is declining, but it remains a critical tool in certain high-risk or complex patients.

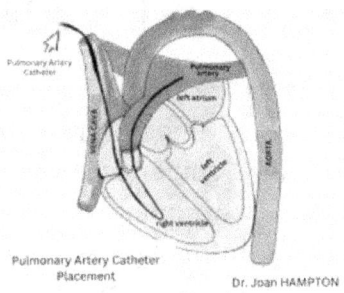

Fig:3.2: Pulmonary Capillary Wedge Pressure Interpretation

SYSTEMIC AND PULMONARY VASCULAR RESISTANCE (SVR AND PVR)

Systemic Vascular Resistance (SVR) and Pulmonary Vascular Resistance (PVR) are key hemodynamic parameters used to assess the resistance that blood encounters as it flows through the body's systemic and pulmonary circulations, respectively. They provide important information about the state of the vascular system and can help diagnose and manage a variety of cardiovascular and pulmonary conditions.

1. What Are SVR and PVR?

- **Systemic Vascular Resistance (SVR)** refers to the resistance that blood faces as it flows through the systemic circulation, primarily determined by the arterioles. SVR is a key factor influencing afterload—the pressure the heart must overcome to pump blood into the arteries.
- **Pulmonary Vascular Resistance (PVR)** is the resistance that blood encounters as it flows through the pulmonary circulation. It reflects the condition of the pulmonary vessels and the pressure the right ventricle must overcome to pump blood through the lungs.

Both parameters are used in critical care to monitor the status of the vascular system and assess the heart's ability to pump blood effectively through the circulations.

2. The Formula for Calculating SVR and PVR

Both SVR and PVR are calculated using standard hemodynamic equations, typically based on mean arterial pressure (MAP) for

SVR, pulmonary artery pressure (PAP) for PVR, and cardiac output (CO).

Systemic Vascular Resistance (SVR) is calculated as:

$SVR = (MAP - CVP)/CO \times 80$

Where:

- MAP = Mean Arterial Pressure
- CVP = Central Venous Pressure
- CO = Cardiac Output
- The constant 80 converts units to dynes·sec·cm^{-5} (the standard unit of resistance)

Pulmonary Vascular Resistance (PVR) is calculated similarly:

$PVR = (MPAP - PCWP)/CO \times 80$

Where:

- MPAP = Mean Pulmonary Artery Pressure
- PCWP = Pulmonary Capillary Wedge Pressure (as a proxy for left atrial pressure)
- CO = Cardiac Output

3. Normal Ranges for SVR and PVR

- **SVR:** The normal range for systemic vascular resistance is **700-1,600 dynes·sec·cm^{-5}**.
- **PVR:** The normal range for pulmonary vascular resistance is **100-250 dynes·sec·cm^{-5}**.

Abnormal values can provide insight into various pathophysiological states affecting the cardiovascular and pulmonary systems.

SVR is an essential parameter in evaluating afterload, which is the resistance the left ventricle must overcome to eject blood into the systemic circulation. Increased SVR can indicate:

- **Hypertension:** Elevated SVR is a hallmark of systemic

hypertension, where the arterioles constrict and increase resistance.
- **Cardiogenic Shock**: In conditions of poor cardiac output, the body may compensate by increasing SVR to maintain blood pressure, which can further burden the heart.
- **Hypovolemic Shock**: In states of significant fluid loss, SVR may increase as the body constricts peripheral vessels to preserve core organ perfusion.
- **Vasoconstriction**: Caused by various factors such as increased sympathetic nervous system activity or the administration of vasopressors, elevated SVR can significantly affect cardiac workload.

5. Clinical Significance of PVR

PVR plays a critical role in assessing the pressure faced by the right ventricle when pumping blood through the pulmonary circulation. Elevated PVR can indicate:

- **Pulmonary Hypertension**: Elevated PVR is a key feature of pulmonary hypertension, a condition where the pulmonary arteries are narrowed or blocked, increasing resistance.
- **Right Ventricular Failure**: As PVR increases, the right ventricle must work harder, potentially leading to right-sided heart failure.
- **Chronic Obstructive Pulmonary Disease (COPD) and Interstitial Lung Disease**: These conditions may result in hypoxic vasoconstriction in the lungs, increasing PVR.

6. Monitoring and Managing Abnormal SVR and PVR

In critically ill patients, monitoring SVR and PVR provides valuable information about the state of their cardiovascular and pulmonary systems, helping guide treatment decisions.

- **High SVR**: When SVR is elevated, treatment is often focused on reducing afterload. This can be achieved using vasodilators such as nitroglycerin or sodium nitroprusside

to reduce the strain on the left ventricle and improve cardiac output.
- **Low SVR**: In conditions such as septic shock, where SVR is abnormally low due to vasodilation, vasopressors like norepinephrine or vasopressin may be used to constrict blood vessels and restore blood pressure.
- **High PVR**: Elevated PVR, as seen in pulmonary hypertension or right heart failure, may be treated with medications such as pulmonary vasodilators (e.g., epoprostenol, sildenafil) to lower pulmonary resistance and improve right ventricular function.
- **Low PVR**: This is typically not a clinical concern but may be noted in conditions where the pulmonary vessels are abnormally dilated.

7. Interpreting SVR and PVR in Clinical Practice

In critical care settings, SVR and PVR are monitored closely, often using invasive techniques like pulmonary artery catheters. By tracking these parameters, clinicians can adjust medications, fluid therapy, and ventilatory support to optimize cardiac function and oxygen delivery.

Examples of Clinical Conditions Affecting SVR and PVR:

- **Increased SVR**: Seen in conditions like **cardiogenic shock, hypovolemia, systemic hypertension**, and when vasopressors are administered.
- **Decreased SVR**: Common in **septic shock, anaphylaxis**, or when vasodilators are used therapeutically.
- **Increased PVR**: Found in **pulmonary hypertension, COPD**, or **ARDS** (Acute Respiratory Distress Syndrome), often necessitating pulmonary-specific treatments.
- **Decreased PVR**: Typically observed in well-oxygenated states or after administration of vasodilators specific to the pulmonary vasculature.

CHAPTER FOUR

Hemodynamic Waveform Analysis

Hemodynamic waveform analysis is a critical component of patient monitoring in intensive care units and other high-acuity settings. Understanding these waveforms allows clinicians to assess the real-time cardiovascular status of their patients, make accurate diagnoses, and implement timely interventions. The dynamic waveforms represent pressure changes within the heart and vessels during the cardiac cycle, offering a visual representation of how well the heart and circulatory system are functioning.

This chapter will guide you through the fundamentals of pressure waveforms, from interpreting arterial and venous waves to recognizing the differences between normal and abnormal patterns. By mastering these concepts, you'll be better equipped to respond to critical changes in a patient's hemodynamic status and troubleshoot any waveform abnormalities or technical artifacts.

Next, we'll explain the specific types of waveforms—arterial, venous, and pulmonary artery pressure wave and explore how they can provide valuable insights into cardiovascular health.

UNDERSTANDING PRESSURE WAVEFORMS

Pressure waveforms are graphical representations of pressure changes within the cardiovascular system, generated by blood flow through the heart and blood vessels. These waveforms provide a real-time view of how the heart is pumping and how blood is moving through the circulatory system. Each waveform has distinct features that reflect the physiological events occurring during the cardiac cycle.

When analyzing pressure waveforms, it is essential to understand the different phases of the cardiac cycle (systole and diastole) and how they correspond to changes in the waveform. Accurately interpreting these waveforms can offer key insights into a patient's hemodynamic status and guide clinical decisions.

1. Components of a Pressure Waveform

- **Upstroke:** The initial rise in the waveform corresponds to ventricular contraction and systole. In arterial waveforms, this reflects the heart pumping blood into the systemic circulation.

- **Peak:** The highest point of the waveform, which represents the maximum pressure exerted during systole.
- **Dicrotic Notch:** This small dip seen in arterial waveforms represents the closure of the aortic valve, marking the transition from systole to diastole.

- **Downstroke:** The decline in the waveform following the peak, which occurs as the heart relaxes and enters diastole. This reflects the decrease in pressure as blood moves away from the heart.

2. Importance of Pressure Waveforms

Pressure waveforms offer valuable information about cardiovascular function. They can be used to assess:

- **Cardiac Output:** The amplitude and shape of the waveform can provide indirect information about how well the heart is pumping blood.
- **Vascular Resistance:** By analyzing the waveform's contours, clinicians can infer the resistance the heart encounters when pumping blood through the circulatory system.
- **Valve Function:** Waveforms can also indicate abnormalities in valve function, such as stenosis or regurgitation, based on characteristic changes in waveform shape.

3. Types of Pressure Waveforms

There are several types of pressure waveforms commonly monitored in critical care, including:

- **Arterial Pressure Waveforms:** Generated from the pressure in major arteries, often used to monitor blood pressure in real-time.
- **Venous Pressure Waveforms:** Reflect the pressure in the veins and the right side of the heart, typically used to assess central venous pressure.
- **Pulmonary Artery Pressure (PAP) Waveforms:** Provide insight into right heart function and pulmonary circulation.

Each type of waveform requires a clear understanding to

ensure proper interpretation and prompt intervention when abnormalities arise.

ARTERIAL, VENOUS, AND PULMONARY ARTERY PRESSURE WAVES

Understanding the various pressure waves—arterial, venous, and pulmonary artery—is essential in monitoring a patient's cardiovascular health. Each type of pressure wave provides unique information about the different areas of the circulatory system. In this section, we'll break down the key characteristics and clinical significance of these waveforms.

1. Arterial Pressure Waveforms

Arterial pressure waveforms are primarily used to continuously monitor systemic blood pressure. These waveforms reflect the pressure exerted by the heart as it pumps blood into the arterial system and are typically recorded via an arterial catheter placed in a major artery (such as the radial or femoral artery).

Key Characteristics:

- **Upstroke**: The rapid rise in the waveform indicates the ventricular contraction (systole), where blood is ejected from the left ventricle into the aorta.
- **Peak (Systolic Pressure)**: The highest point on the waveform represents the systolic pressure—the maximum pressure exerted on the arterial walls during heart contraction.
- **Dicrotic Notch**: This small dip occurs after the peak and marks the closure of the aortic valve, signaling the end of systole and the beginning of diastole.
- **Downstroke (Diastolic Pressure)**: The gradual decline

represents the relaxation of the ventricles and the decrease in arterial pressure as the heart refills with blood.

Clinical Relevance:

- Arterial pressure waveforms are crucial in detecting hypotension, hypertension, and pulse pressure variations.
- The dicrotic notch serves as an indicator of proper aortic valve function.

2. Venous Pressure Waveforms

Venous pressure waveforms are generated by the pressure in the central veins (commonly from the superior vena cava) and reflect the pressure dynamics of the right atrium and right ventricle. Central venous pressure (CVP) monitoring provides insight into a patient's fluid status and right heart function.

Key Components:

- **A Wave**: Represents atrial contraction, typically occurring just after the P wave on the ECG.
- **C Wave**: A small, upward deflection seen during ventricular contraction (systole), caused by the closure of the tricuspid valve and subsequent bulging into the atrium.
- **V Wave**: Occurs as the atrium fills during ventricular systole and peaks just before the opening of the tricuspid valve for the next diastolic phase.

Clinical Relevance:

- Elevated CVP waveforms may indicate fluid overload, right heart failure, or pulmonary hypertension.
- Abnormal venous waveforms can reveal tricuspid regurgitation or arrhythmias.

3. Pulmonary Artery Pressure (PAP) Waveforms

Pulmonary artery pressure waveforms are used to monitor the pressure in the pulmonary artery and provide insight into the function of the right side of the heart and pulmonary circulation. This is commonly measured with a pulmonary artery catheter (also known as a Swan-Ganz catheter).

Key Features:

- **Systolic Pressure (PAS):** The peak of the pulmonary artery waveform represents the systolic pressure, reflecting right ventricular contraction.
- **Diastolic Pressure (PAD):** The lower point of the waveform represents the diastolic pressure, measured as the right ventricle fills with blood.
- **Pulmonary Capillary Wedge Pressure (PCWP):** This is measured when the catheter balloon inflates in the pulmonary artery, indirectly reflecting left atrial pressure.

Clinical Relevance:

- PAP waveforms are critical for diagnosing pulmonary hypertension and assessing right ventricular function.
- PCWP helps assess left-sided heart function and can indicate left ventricular failure or mitral valve disease.

Recognizing Normal vs. Abnormal Waveforms

One of the key skills in hemodynamic monitoring is the ability to differentiate between normal and abnormal waveforms. Normal waveforms reflect proper cardiovascular function, while abnormal waveforms can signal a variety of clinical issues, including heart failure, valve dysfunction, and vascular resistance problems. Early recognition of these abnormalities is crucial for timely intervention and effective patient care.

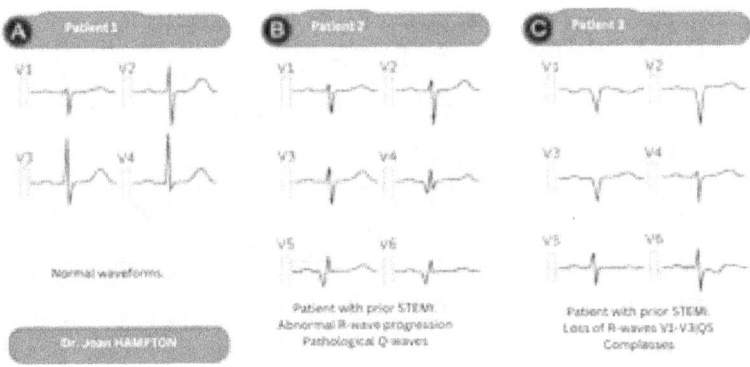

Fig 4.1: Normal and Abnormal waveforms

1. Normal Waveforms

A normal pressure waveform typically exhibits consistent, predictable patterns that correspond with the phases of the cardiac cycle. Here's a breakdown of what to expect from normal waveforms for different monitoring types:

Normal Arterial Waveform

- **Upstroke**: Rapid, sharp rise due to ventricular systole.
- **Peak (Systolic Pressure)**: High point of the waveform.
- **Dicrotic Notch**: Represents aortic valve closure, a key indicator of a healthy cardiac cycle.
- **Downstroke**: Smooth descent during diastole as the ventricles relax.

Clinical Implications:

- A normal arterial waveform indicates adequate cardiac output and proper valve function.

Normal Venous Waveform (CVP)

- **A Wave**: Slight rise during atrial contraction.
- **C Wave**: Small upward deflection during ventricular systole, caused by the bulging of the tricuspid valve.
- **V Wave**: Gradual rise during atrial filling, followed by a rapid drop as the tricuspid valve opens.

Clinical Implications:

- A normal CVP waveform suggests healthy right heart function and fluid balance.

Normal Pulmonary Artery Pressure (PAP) Waveform

- **Systolic Wave:** Represents right ventricular contraction, with a peak corresponding to pulmonary artery systolic pressure.
- **Diastolic Wave:** Represents right ventricular relaxation and pulmonary artery diastolic pressure.

Clinical Implications:

- Normal PAP waveforms reflect proper pulmonary circulation and right ventricular function.

2. Abnormal Waveforms

Abnormal waveforms may appear due to various cardiovascular conditions. Identifying these abnormalities is essential for diagnosing underlying issues and adjusting treatment accordingly.

Abnormal Arterial Waveforms

- **Flattened or Blunted Waveform:** Indicates low stroke volume, which may be caused by hypovolemia, heart failure, or severe aortic stenosis.
- **Absent Dicrotic Notch:** Can suggest aortic regurgitation or low systemic vascular resistance.
- **Spiked or Slurred Upstroke:** May indicate hypertrophic cardiomyopathy or other forms of obstruction to blood flow.

Clinical Implications:

- These waveforms can indicate impaired cardiac output or vascular resistance problems, requiring prompt intervention.

Abnormal Venous Waveforms (CVP)

- **Elevated A Waves (Cannon A Waves):** Seen with atrioventricular dissociation (e.g., complete heart block), where the atrium contracts against a closed tricuspid valve.
- **Prominent V Waves:** Often associated with tricuspid regurgitation, where blood flows back into the atrium during systole, creating large V waves.
- **Absence of A or V Waves:** This can be seen in atrial fibrillation, where the loss of organized atrial contraction leads to absent or abnormal waves.

Clinical Implications:

- Abnormal CVP waveforms suggest issues with atrial contraction, tricuspid valve function, or arrhythmias.

Abnormal Pulmonary Artery Pressure (PAP) Waveforms

- **Elevated Systolic Pressure:** May indicate pulmonary hypertension, where increased resistance in the pulmonary circulation causes high systolic pressure.
- **Elevated Diastolic Pressure:** Can suggest left ventricular failure or mitral valve disease, as blood backs up into the pulmonary circulation.
- **Absent or Flattened Waveform:** May result from catheter misplacement or technical issues, requiring recalibration or catheter repositioning.

Clinical Implications:

- Abnormal PAP waveforms signal potential issues in the pulmonary circulation or right-sided heart failure.

CLINICAL PRACTICE TIP:

When recognizing abnormal waveforms:

- Always check for calibration errors or catheter malposition before diagnosing a clinical issue.
- Correlate waveform changes with the patient's overall clinical condition (e.g., vital signs, lab results, symptoms).

By mastering the ability to recognize abnormal waveforms, clinicians can intervene earlier and improve patient outcomes in critical situations.

TROUBLESHOOTING ARTIFACTS AND ABNORMALITIES

In hemodynamic monitoring, artifacts and abnormalities can interfere with waveform readings, potentially leading to misinterpretation of a patient's status. Recognizing and resolving these issues is essential for accurate monitoring and optimal patient care. This section will address common sources of artifacts and abnormalities in hemodynamic waveforms, from equipment-related issues to physiological causes, and provide practical troubleshooting strategies.

1. Identify the Source of Artifact

Artifacts can stem from mechanical issues, patient movement, electrical interference, or improper setup of monitoring equipment. For instance, loose connections or air bubbles in catheter lines often cause erroneous readings. First, confirm that all equipment is securely connected, properly calibrated, and free of air bubbles.

2. Observe Consistency and Symmetry

Normal waveforms display consistent shapes and patterns. Inconsistent waveform shapes, erratic peaks, or changes in amplitude might indicate an artifact. Comparing waveforms across multiple monitoring sites (if applicable) can help confirm abnormalities versus artifacts.

3. Eliminate Common Mechanical Artifacts

Mechanical issues are frequent causes of waveform

irregularities. Look for kinks in lines, improperly zeroed transducers, or excessive catheter length, which can create damping effects. Adjust catheter positioning as needed to restore normal waveform appearance.

4. Patient Movement or Positioning Issues

Patient movement, including coughing or changing position, can distort waveforms. When sudden waveform changes occur, assess whether the patient's movement may be the cause. Reposition or stabilize the patient if needed, and allow waveforms to settle.

5. Recognize and Correct Electrical Interference

Interference from other electronic devices or static can disrupt waveforms. Ensure that monitoring cables and equipment are free from direct contact with other devices. Additionally, the grounding of electrical equipment in the monitoring area must be assessed.

CHAPTER FIVE

Step-by-Step Guide to Invasive Hemodynamic Monitoring

For critically ill patients, hemodynamic monitoring and intervention techniques are crucial to assess and stabilize cardiovascular function. This chapter focuses on essential procedures used to measure and optimize hemodynamic parameters, providing a foundation for effective patient management in acute and critical care settings. Techniques such as arterial line insertion, central venous catheterization, pulmonary artery catheterization, and dynamic assessments are each invaluable in specific contexts, allowing for precise monitoring and responsive treatment.

In this chapter, we will cover:

- **Arterial Lines:** Insertion, management, and troubleshooting for accurate blood pressure monitoring and frequent blood sampling.
- **Central Venous Catheters:** Indications, placement methods, and management protocols to facilitate central venous pressure measurements and medication delivery.
- **Pulmonary Artery Catheterization:** Techniques and rationale for using pulmonary artery catheters to measure complex cardiovascular parameters.
- **Dynamic Assessments:** Evaluating fluid responsiveness through passive leg raise and fluid challenge techniques, which help guide resuscitation efforts and optimize volume status.

By understanding these methods, clinical staff will be equipped to enhance patient outcomes through precise monitoring and responsive intervention.

CENTRAL VENOUS CATHETERS: PLACEMENT AND MANAGEMENT

Central venous catheters (CVCs) play a critical role in patient care, particularly in intensive care units (ICUs) and surgical settings, by providing access for medications, fluids, and hemodynamic monitoring. A CVC is typically inserted into large veins, such as the internal jugular, subclavian, or femoral vein, allowing access to the central circulation. Proper placement, management, and understanding of potential complications are crucial for healthcare providers working with CVCs.

Indications for Central Venous Catheter Placement

CVCs are commonly indicated in patients who need:

- **Hemodynamic Monitoring**: CVCs allow for measurement of central venous pressure (CVP), which assists in evaluating fluid status and cardiac function.
- **Rapid Infusion of Fluids or Blood Products**: In cases of significant fluid loss, shock, or sepsis.
- **Medication Administration**: CVCs provide access for vasoactive medications, chemotherapy, and other drugs that may irritate smaller veins.
- **Long-term IV Therapy**: Ideal for patients who require extended IV access or parenteral nutrition.

Preparation and Required Equipment

A sterile environment and the following equipment are essential:

- CVC kit (including guidewire, dilator, and catheter)
- Ultrasound (for guided insertion to improve accuracy and reduce complications)
- Sterile drapes, gloves, and antiseptics
- Suture materials and securement devices

Note: Ultrasound guidance is recommended for CVC placement as it enhances accuracy and reduces complications, especially in high-risk patients.

Placement Technique

1. **Patient Positioning and Preparation**: Position the patient to ensure vein accessibility, typically in Trendelenburg position for jugular or subclavian access.
2. **Site Selection**: Choose the appropriate vein based on the patient's condition and access needs, with preference for the internal jugular or subclavian in most settings due to lower infection rates.
3. **Aseptic Insertion**:
    - **Sterile Field**: Ensure a sterile field and aseptic technique.
    - **Local Anesthesia**: Apply local anesthetic at the insertion site.
    - **Catheter Insertion**: Use the Seldinger technique, advancing a guidewire into the vein, followed by catheter placement over the guidewire.
    - **Securement**: Once the catheter is placed, secure it with sutures or securement devices to minimize movement.
4. **Post-insertion Care**: Confirm placement with imaging (usually a chest X-ray) to ensure proper positioning and absence of complications, such as pneumothorax.

Management and Maintenance

Effective maintenance is essential for preventing catheter-related bloodstream infections (CRBSIs) and other complications:

- **Sterile Dressing Changes**: Regularly change dressings using sterile technique.
- **Line Patency and Flushes**: Flush the line with saline to maintain patency, avoiding air embolism or clotting.
- **Daily Assessment**: Assess the need for the catheter daily to minimize the risk of infection.

Troubleshooting Common Issues

- **Catheter Occlusion**: Check the line for kinks or blood clots and consider using clot-dissolving agents if necessary.
- **Infection**: Monitor for signs of infection at the insertion site, including redness, swelling, and discharge, and follow strict protocols for aseptic dressing changes.
- **Mechanical Complications**: Recognize complications such as pneumothorax, hematoma, or arterial puncture, especially during or immediately after placement.

Both the PLR and Fluid Challenge are invaluable in assessing fluid responsiveness and preventing unnecessary fluid overload, ultimately improving patient outcomes in critical care.

PULMONARY ARTERY CATHETERIZATION TECHNIQUES

Pulmonary artery catheterization (PAC), also known as Swan-Ganz catheterization, is a procedure used to measure hemodynamic variables that help guide the management of critically ill patients. By directly measuring pressures within the heart and pulmonary artery, PAC provides data on cardiac function, preload, afterload, and overall circulatory health. Although PAC has become less common due to less invasive alternatives, it remains invaluable in certain complex cases.

INDICATIONS FOR PULMONARY ARTERY CATHETERIZATION

PAC is often reserved for patients in whom detailed hemodynamic assessment is critical, such as those with:

- **Severe Heart Failure**: Where monitoring cardiac output and pressures is essential.
- **Complex Shock States**: To differentiate between hypovolemic, cardiogenic, and distributive shock.
- **Pulmonary Hypertension**: PAC helps assess the extent of the condition and monitor the response to treatments.
- **Severe Acute Respiratory Distress Syndrome (ARDS)**: To guide fluid management.

PROCEDURE PREPARATION AND EQUIPMENT

Performing PAC requires meticulous preparation to ensure safety and accuracy:

- **Equipment**: A Swan-Ganz catheter, central venous access setup, monitoring equipment for continuous waveform display, and a sterile kit.
- **Aseptic Field**: The procedure should be carried out under strict aseptic conditions to prevent infection.
- **Sedation and Positioning**: Light sedation may be administered, and the patient should be positioned to maximize vein accessibility, often supine.

INSERTION TECHNIQUE

1. **Central Venous Access**: PAC requires central venous access, typically achieved through the internal jugular or subclavian vein.
2. **Catheter Advancement**:
   - **Right Atrium**: The catheter is advanced into the right atrium, where the first waveform appears on the monitor.
   - **Right Ventricle**: Advancing the catheter further reaches the right ventricle, producing a characteristic waveform.
   - **Pulmonary Artery**: As the catheter progresses, it enters the pulmonary artery, revealing a distinct waveform pattern.
   - **Pulmonary Capillary Wedge Position**: By further advancing, the catheter can "wedge" into a smaller pulmonary artery branch, allowing for measurement of pulmonary capillary wedge pressure (PCWP).
3. **Monitoring and Waveform Recognition**: The catheter is advanced while observing pressure waveforms on the monitor to confirm its position at each stage of the procedure.

MEASUREMENTS AND DATA INTERPRETATION

The PAC provides crucial data including:

- **Pulmonary Artery Pressure (PAP)**: Helps assess the state of the pulmonary circulation.
- **Pulmonary Capillary Wedge Pressure (PCWP)**: Estimates left atrial pressure, informing on left heart function and fluid status.
- **Cardiac Output (CO)**: Derived from thermodilution or the Fick principle, CO measurements are central to managing hemodynamic stability.

RISKS AND COMPLICATIONS

While PAC can provide essential data, it is associated with certain risks:

- **Arrhythmias**: Especially ventricular arrhythmias during catheter advancement through the heart.
- **Pulmonary Artery Rupture**: A rare but serious complication.
- **Infection**: Strict sterile techniques are essential to minimize infection risks.
- **Thromboembolism**: Prolonged catheter presence may increase the risk of clots.

Pulmonary artery catheterization remains a sophisticated tool in managing hemodynamically unstable patients, and it requires a well-trained team to perform the procedure safely and accurately.

DYNAMIC ASSESSMENTS: PASSIVE LEG RAISE, FLUID CHALLENGE

Dynamic assessments are crucial in hemodynamic monitoring to evaluate a patient's fluid responsiveness, which helps guide fluid management in critical care. Two primary methods for this are the Passive Leg Raise (PLR) and the Fluid Challenge. Both are non-invasive techniques used to assess whether a patient would benefit from additional fluids or if they're at risk of fluid overload. Each test provides important data on the patient's cardiovascular status without the immediate need for administering large fluid volumes.

Passive Leg Raise (PLR)

The Passive Leg Raise is a reversible, bedside maneuver that acts as an "internal fluid challenge" by temporarily shifting venous blood from the lower extremities to the central circulation, effectively increasing preload and mimicking a small fluid bolus.

Procedure:

- Place the patient in a semi-recumbent position.
- Raise both legs passively to about 45 degrees.
- Monitor changes in cardiac output or stroke volume within 30–90 seconds.

Interpretation:

Positive Response: An increase in cardiac output (typically >10-15%) suggests the patient may benefit from fluid administration.

Negative Response: Little to no change in cardiac output indicates that fluid administration may not improve hemodynamic status and could risk overload.

Clinical Importance: The PLR test is simple, repeatable, and safe, providing a temporary preload increase without additional fluid, making it ideal for patients where fluid status is challenging to assess.

Fluid Challenge

A Fluid Challenge is a controlled administration of a small fluid bolus to observe hemodynamic changes in response. It is used to confirm if a patient is fluid-responsive and can tolerate fluid infusion.

Procedure:

- Administer a small bolus (e.g., 250–500 mL of isotonic crystalloid solution) over a short period (5–10 minutes).
- Monitor hemodynamic parameters, such as cardiac output or stroke volume, before and after administration.

Interpretation:

Positive Response: A marked increase in cardiac output or stroke volume suggests the patient can benefit from additional fluid administration.

Negative Response: Minimal or no change may indicate that the patient has reached adequate or excess fluid levels and should not receive more fluids.

Clinical Importance: The fluid challenge is especially useful in settings where precise fluid management is essential but is contraindicated in cases of volume overload or heart failure.

When it comes to evaluating fluid responsiveness and avoiding needless fluid overload, the PLR and Fluid Challenge are both quite helpful in enhancing patient outcomes in critical care.

CHAPTER SIX

Non-Invasive Hemodynamic Monitoring

Advancements in non-invasive hemodynamic monitoring have transformed critical care, allowing clinicians to assess cardiovascular function with reduced risk and increased patient comfort. Non-invasive methods like **Doppler Ultrasound**, **Echocardiography**, and **Pulse Contour Analysis** provide detailed hemodynamic data without requiring catheterization or other invasive approaches, making them especially useful in cases where traditional methods may be contraindicated or difficult to implement.

These tools not only provide vital information on parameters like cardiac output, stroke volume, and vascular resistance but also allow for real-time monitoring. As technology continues to evolve, newer, advanced non-invasive techniques are enhancing accuracy and applicability across a wide range of patient settings, from intensive care units to operating rooms and emergency departments.

The main non-invasive hemodynamic monitoring techniques are examined in this chapter, with an emphasis on how they work, their advantages, disadvantages, and how they aid in clinical decision-making. The basic ideas of Doppler Ultrasound and Echocardiography will be covered first, followed by an examination of the procedure and interpretation of Pulse Contour Analysis and a summary of cutting-edge non-invasive methods that could expand the use of hemodynamic monitoring.

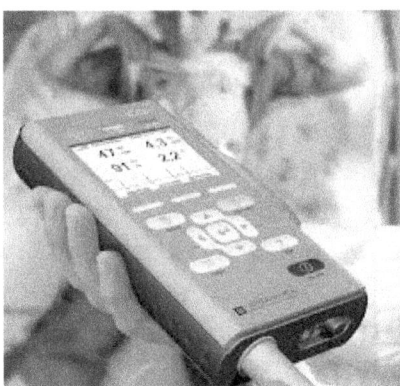

Fig 6.1: Non-invasive treatment

Doppler Ultrasound and Echocardiography

Doppler Ultrasound and **Echocardiography** are fundamental non-invasive tools for evaluating hemodynamic function, frequently used in clinical and critical care settings. These methods rely on sound waves to visualize and assess the cardiovascular system's structure and function, enabling accurate and real-time insights into blood flow, cardiac output, and vascular resistance. Here's how each tool contributes to hemodynamic monitoring:

DOPPLER ULTRASOUND

Doppler Ultrasound utilizes the Doppler effect to measure blood flow velocity in vessels. As sound waves are emitted by the transducer, they reflect off moving blood cells, and the changes in frequency allow clinicians to calculate blood flow velocity and direction.

Uses:

- Assessment of blood flow in major arteries and veins.
- Estimation of cardiac output by calculating flow velocity across specific points in the heart.
- Measurement of vascular resistance to aid in evaluating circulatory efficiency.

Advantages:

- Safe and highly accessible with minimal preparation.
- Provides continuous and real-time monitoring, especially useful for cardiac patients and those in critical care.

Limitations:

- Dependent on the skill of the operator for accuracy.
- Limited in cases where acoustic windows are difficult to obtain, such as in patients with obesity or certain anatomical variations.

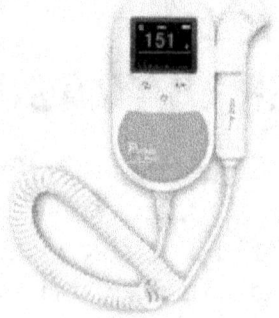

Fig 6.2: Droppler

ECHOCARDIOGRAPHY

Echocardiography, commonly referred to as "echo," goes a step further by providing two-dimensional images of the heart. Using high-frequency sound waves, echocardiography produces detailed visuals of the heart's chambers, valves, and surrounding structures, making it invaluable for assessing cardiac function and anatomy.

Types of Echocardiography:

1. **Transthoracic Echocardiography (TTE):** A standard, external approach where the transducer is placed on the chest wall to obtain images.
2. **Transesophageal Echocardiography (TEE):** Invasive but highly effective, TEE involves inserting the transducer into the esophagus to get clearer images of the heart's posterior structures.

Uses:

- Evaluation of cardiac chamber size, wall thickness, and ejection fraction.
- Detection of valve abnormalities, pericardial effusions, and congenital heart defects.
- Measurement of stroke volume and cardiac output, which are critical in assessing hemodynamic status.

Advantages:

- Provides a detailed view of heart structure and motion.
- Useful for both structural assessment and functional measurement, making it an essential tool in cardiovascular diagnostics.

Limitations:

- TTE may be limited by poor acoustic windows in certain patients, requiring TEE.
- TEE, while providing better image clarity, is more invasive and not always practical.

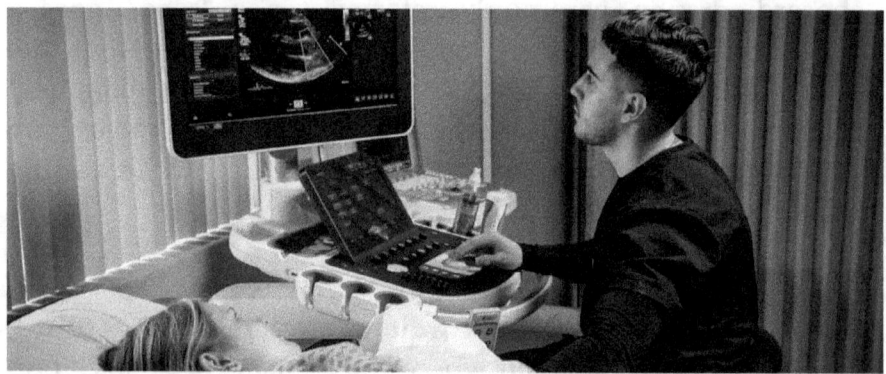

Fig 6.3: Echocardiography been used for a patient

Both echocardiography and Doppler ultrasound are essential for non-invasive hemodynamic monitoring because they offer complimentary information that helps create a comprehensive picture of cardiovascular health. Clinicians can choose the best instrument for their patients' particular needs by being aware of each one's advantages and disadvantages.

PULSE CONTOUR ANALYSIS

Pulse Contour Analysis (PCA) is an advanced method in hemodynamic monitoring that enables continuous measurement of cardiac output (CO) and stroke volume (SV) through analysis of the arterial pulse waveform. This non-invasive, real-time approach allows for dynamic assessments of hemodynamic status without requiring invasive techniques such as pulmonary artery catheterization.

How Pulse Contour Analysis Works

Pulse Contour Analysis interprets the morphology of the arterial pulse waveform, which changes based on the stroke volume ejected from the heart and the compliance of the arterial system. By examining the area under the systolic portion of the waveform, PCA algorithms can estimate stroke volume, and from this, cardiac output can be calculated. Some systems also combine PCA with additional calibration techniques, such as transpulmonary thermodilution, to improve accuracy.

1. **Arterial Line Required**: An arterial catheter, usually placed in the radial artery, is required to capture the pressure waveforms. The waveform data is then analyzed by a PCA device or monitoring system.
2. **Continuous Monitoring**: PCA provides a continuous stream of data on cardiac output, stroke volume, and other hemodynamic parameters, offering a dynamic view of changes over time.
3. **Algorithm Calibration**: While uncalibrated systems can provide real-time data, calibrated systems that adjust for patient-specific variables (like vascular tone and compliance) are more accurate.

APPLICATIONS OF PULSE CONTOUR ANALYSIS

PCA is frequently utilized in emergency rooms, critical care units, and surgical settings, especially for hemodynamically unstable patients. Fluid management benefits greatly from the continuous data it offers, which can be used to guide interventions such as fluid administration or medication modifications based on real-time responses.

- **Fluid Responsiveness**: PCA helps clinicians assess fluid responsiveness through parameters like Stroke Volume Variation (SVV) or Pulse Pressure Variation (PPV), which indicate if a patient is likely to benefit from additional fluids.
- **Vasopressor Therapy Monitoring**: In patients receiving vasopressors, PCA assists in tracking cardiac output to ensure optimal blood flow and perfusion.
- **Guiding Perioperative Care**: PCA is useful during major surgeries for monitoring hemodynamic parameters continuously, enabling immediate interventions if instability is detected.

BENEFITS AND LIMITATIONS OF PULSE CONTOUR ANALYSIS

Benefits:

- **Non-Invasive to Minimally Invasive**: Compared to traditional cardiac output measurements that may involve central venous or pulmonary artery catheterization, PCA is significantly less invasive.
- **Real-Time Data**: Provides instantaneous feedback, essential for monitoring hemodynamic trends and making rapid adjustments.
- **Dynamic Measurements**: Especially useful for assessing fluid responsiveness and adjusting therapy in critically ill patients.

Limitations:

- **Arterial Catheter Requirement**: Requires an arterial line, which, while less invasive than some methods, is still not without risks (e.g., infection, arterial injury).
- **Accuracy Variability**: PCA's accuracy can be influenced by patient-specific factors such as vascular compliance, arrhythmias, and extreme hemodynamic changes. Calibrated PCA systems, which require initial or periodic calibration with another CO measurement technique, are generally more accurate.

In complex clinical settings, pulse contour analysis is a vital technique for continuous, non-invasive hemodynamic monitoring. Clinicians can improve patient outcomes in critical and perioperative care by making well-informed, real-time decisions based on their grasp of waveform data and its uses.

ADVANCED NON-INVASIVE TECHNIQUES

Recent developments in medical technology have made it possible to do hemodynamic monitoring using a number of non-invasive techniques that offer thorough, real-time cardiovascular data without invasive catheterization. These methods provide quicker, safer evaluations, which are particularly helpful in outpatient situations or for patients for whom intrusive monitoring presents serious dangers. We'll look at some of the most popular cutting-edge non-invasive methods here.

Common Advanced Non-Invasive Hemodynamic Monitoring Techniques

1. **Bioreactance Technology**
   - Bioreactance is a relatively new technology that measures blood flow based on phase shifts that occur as an electrical current passes through the thorax. This technology allows for continuous monitoring of cardiac output and other hemodynamic parameters.
   - It is highly beneficial in critical care and perioperative environments where rapid changes in cardiac output need to be monitored, and it does not require an arterial line, unlike many other monitoring methods.
2. **Impedance Cardiography (ICG)**
   - ICG is a method that measures changes in thoracic electrical impedance, which vary with blood flow in the chest. This technique is used to measure cardiac output, stroke volume, and systemic vascular resistance in real-time.

- ICG is particularly useful in settings like intensive care units and emergency departments, as it provides real-time cardiac data without the invasiveness of catheter-based monitoring.

3. **Pulse Transit Time (PTT) Monitoring**
- PTT uses the time taken for a blood pulse to travel between two arterial sites to estimate blood pressure and cardiac output. This technology has found applications in wearable health technology and portable monitoring devices.
- It is ideal for patients needing continuous blood pressure monitoring over extended periods, and it has significant potential for remote and ambulatory monitoring.

4. **Photoplethysmography (PPG)**
- PPG uses light to measure blood volume changes in the microvascular bed of tissue, offering valuable data on pulse rate, oxygen saturation, and heart rate variability. Although it primarily provides peripheral information, PPG is being integrated with machine learning algorithms to improve its accuracy in estimating central hemodynamic parameters.
- It is commonly used in settings that require frequent monitoring without invasive access, like outpatient clinics and monitoring during physical activity or in remote environments.

APPLICATIONS AND ADVANTAGES

Each of these methods provides benefits by offering hemodynamic data without the need for invasive access. They allow for continuous, real-time data acquisition, reducing the need for catheterization and lowering the risk of complications like infections or arterial injuries.

Benefits:

- **Minimized Patient Risk**: Lowered infection and complication rates as compared to invasive methods.
- **Ease of Use**: Can often be set up quickly and with minimal training, which is crucial in emergency settings.
- **Mobility**: Non-invasive systems allow for better mobility, which is beneficial in rehabilitation settings, at-home care, or for patients on the move.

Limitations:

- **Accuracy in Specific Populations**: In cases of arrhythmias or other cardiovascular abnormalities, some non-invasive techniques may provide less accurate data than invasive methods.
- **Sensitivity to Movement**: Certain methods, like PPG and PTT, may be affected by patient movement, impacting data quality during physical activity.

Non-invasive hemodynamic monitoring, which provides safer, simpler, and more pleasant monitoring choices for a variety of clinical settings, is a major advancement in patient care.

Without utilizing intrusive techniques, physicians can obtain precise hemodynamic data by utilizing Doppler ultrasound, pulse contour analysis, and cutting-edge technologies like bioreactance and impedance cardiography. From outpatient management to acute critical care, each instrument has special benefits that are appropriate for various patient circumstances and clinical requirements.

Non-invasive methods may not always be as accurate as intrusive monitoring, especially in complex or high-risk cases, even while they lower the risk of infection, minimize patient discomfort, and enable faster adoption. Effective hemodynamic assessment still depends on the clinician's ability to choose and interpret the right non-invasive instruments. Non-invasive techniques will probably become even more accurate and useful as technology develops, improving patient outcomes and developing the area of hemodynamic monitoring in the process.

An overview of the primary non-invasive instruments has been given in this chapter, giving you the fundamental knowledge you need to incorporate these methods into clinical practice and enhance patient comfort and safety.

CHAPTER SEVEN

Hemodynamic Assessment for Different Clinical Scenarios

Hemodynamic monitoring is crucial for managing patients across a spectrum of clinical conditions, as it helps guide treatment decisions and predict patient outcomes. Each scenario presents unique hemodynamic challenges, requiring an understanding of specific parameters and monitoring techniques to maintain stability and optimize patient care.

This chapter explores hemodynamic assessment in several key situations: managing hypotension and shock, monitoring changes in sepsis and cardiogenic shock, assessing patients with heart failure, and addressing hemodynamic needs in post-operative care. By examining these clinical contexts, we will discuss practical monitoring strategies and adjustments that enhance patient outcomes, whether the goal is to stabilize blood pressure, maintain adequate organ perfusion, or manage fluid balance.

This chapter aims to give healthcare professionals the information they need to enhance bedside decision-making and apply hemodynamic principles to a variety of clinical settings, many of which are difficult. It does this by providing insights specific to certain scenarios.

Managing Hypotension and Shock

Hypotension, or low blood pressure, is a critical sign often associated with shock, a life-threatening condition where blood flow to organs is inadequate to meet metabolic needs. Proper management requires understanding the underlying cause of the shock, as each type—hypovolemic, cardiogenic, distributive, and obstructive—has distinct hemodynamic profiles and treatment strategies.

1. **Assessing the Type of Shock**:
   - In **hypovolemic shock** (e.g., from blood loss or dehydration), there is a marked reduction in blood volume, which decreases preload and cardiac output. Treatment involves volume resuscitation to restore circulating blood volume.
   - **Cardiogenic shock** occurs when the heart's pumping ability is compromised, often due to myocardial infarction or severe heart failure. Here, preload may increase, but cardiac output is impaired, requiring careful management with inotropes to support heart function without worsening the volume overload.
   - **Distributive shock**, commonly caused by sepsis, features widespread vasodilation that leads to low systemic vascular resistance (SVR) and pooling of blood in the periphery. Fluid resuscitation and vasopressors help increase blood pressure and perfusion.
   - In **obstructive shock** (e.g., pulmonary embolism or tension pneumothorax), blood flow is mechanically restricted, requiring interventions that address the obstruction directly (e.g., anticoagulation or relieving pressure).

2. **Hemodynamic Monitoring in Shock**:
   - **Mean Arterial Pressure (MAP)**: Maintaining MAP above 65 mmHg is often a therapeutic goal to ensure adequate organ perfusion.
   - **Central Venous Pressure (CVP)** and **Pulmonary Capillary Wedge Pressure (PCWP)**: These measurements help assess preload, especially in

hypovolemic and cardiogenic shock.
- **Cardiac Output (CO)** and **Cardiac Index (CI)**: Monitoring CO and CI aids in determining if cardiac function is sufficient and guiding inotropic therapy, especially in cardiogenic shock.
- **Systemic Vascular Resistance (SVR)**: SVR provides insights into vascular tone, which is crucial in distributive shock management.

3. **Therapeutic Interventions**:
- **Fluids**: Fluid resuscitation is often the first step in hypovolemic and distributive shock but must be carefully monitored in cardiogenic shock.
- **Vasoactive Medications**: Vasopressors like norepinephrine are typically used to maintain blood pressure in distributive shock, while inotropes such as dobutamine support cardiac output in cardiogenic shock.
- **Advanced Interventions**: For cases like obstructive shock, thrombolytic therapy or surgical intervention may be necessary.

Hemodynamic monitoring and customized therapies must be carefully combined to manage hypotension and shock. In order to direct fluid therapy, pharmaceutical administration, and sophisticated interventions that finally stabilize the patient and restore perfusion to critical organs, it is imperative to comprehend the hemodynamic alterations that are specific to each kind of shock.

HEMODYNAMIC CHANGES IN SEPSIS AND CARDIOGENIC SHOCK

Despite having different hemodynamic characteristics, sepsis and cardiogenic shock can both result in severe hemodynamic instability. Comprehending these profiles is crucial for directing suitable treatment measures to bolster organ function and restore stability.

HEMODYNAMIC PROFILE OF SEPSIS

In sepsis, an infection triggers a systemic inflammatory response that leads to widespread vasodilation, capillary leakage, and increased vascular permeability. These processes result in:

1. **Decreased Systemic Vascular Resistance (SVR)**: As blood vessels dilate, SVR falls, leading to hypotension and inadequate organ perfusion.
2. **Increased Cardiac Output (CO)** (initially): The heart may reflexively boost CO to make up for decreased SVR. Known as "hyperdynamic sepsis," this initial stage is frequently characterized by tachycardia and a warm periphery brought on by vasodilation.
3. **Hypotension**: Despite the elevated CO, blood pressure remains low due to decreased SVR, requiring vasopressors like norepinephrine to help maintain adequate MAP.
4. **Reduced Preload**: Capillary leakage can lead to a drop in intravascular volume, reducing preload. This can further complicate hemodynamic management, especially in later stages of sepsis.

Monitoring Considerations:

- **CVP and MAP**: Monitoring these helps guide fluid resuscitation to maintain adequate preload and perfusion.
- **Cardiac Index (CI)**: Elevated CI indicates the hyperdynamic state in early sepsis, while a drop can signify worsening sepsis.

- **Lactate Levels**: An indirect measure of perfusion, elevated lactate suggests tissue hypoxia and helps guide the aggressiveness of resuscitation efforts.

HEMODYNAMIC PROFILE OF CARDIOGENIC SHOCK

Cardiogenic shock, typically resulting from severe myocardial infarction or heart failure, reflects the heart's inability to pump effectively. Unlike sepsis, cardiogenic shock is characterized by:

1. **Reduced Cardiac Output (CO)**: The heart's decreased pumping ability leads to lower CO and CI, impairing perfusion and oxygen delivery to tissues.
2. **Increased Systemic Vascular Resistance (SVR)**: As CO drops, the body compensates with vasoconstriction to maintain MAP. This increased SVR, however, adds to the workload of an already compromised heart.
3. **Elevated Preload**: Due to poor ventricular emptying, preload (measured by CVP or PCWP) increases, which can lead to pulmonary congestion and worsening heart failure symptoms.
4. **Hypotension**: Persistent hypotension, despite vasoconstriction, indicates severe left ventricular dysfunction and may require inotropic support.

Monitoring Considerations:

- **MAP and PCWP**: Both are vital for assessing fluid status and guiding interventions like diuretics or vasopressors.
- **Pulmonary Artery Catheterization**: Can help monitor left and right ventricular function and differentiate cardiogenic from other types of shock.
- **Oxygen Saturation and SvO2**: Low values can indicate inadequate tissue oxygenation, guiding inotropic support or fluid adjustments.

MANAGEMENT IMPLICATIONS

- **Sepsis**: In early sepsis, aggressive fluid resuscitation is crucial to maintain preload and MAP, but excessive fluids should be avoided as sepsis progresses. Vasopressors, particularly norepinephrine, are often required to increase SVR and maintain perfusion.
- **Cardiogenic Shock**: Management focuses on supporting cardiac output while avoiding excessive fluid overload. Inotropes, like dobutamine, improve myocardial contractility, while careful diuresis can relieve pulmonary congestion. Mechanical support devices (e.g., intra-aortic balloon pump) may be considered in severe cases.

For the purpose of directing therapies that target the distinct hemodynamic abnormalities found in sepsis and cardiogenic shock, hemodynamic monitoring is crucial in both situations. In these intricate critical care situations, clinicians can enhance patient outcomes by customizing treatment to the underlying hemodynamic demands, whether that be restoring SVR in sepsis or sustaining CO in cardiogenic shock.

Monitoring in Patients with Heart Failure

In heart failure (HF), effective hemodynamic monitoring is essential to assess cardiac function, guide treatment, and improve patient outcomes. Heart failure results from the heart's inability to pump sufficient blood to meet the body's demands, leading to fluid overload, reduced cardiac output, and tissue hypoxia. Monitoring provides real-time insights into the heart's performance and helps clinicians adjust therapies to alleviate symptoms and optimize heart function.

KEY HEMODYNAMIC PARAMETERS IN HEART FAILURE

1. **Central Venous Pressure (CVP)**: CVP monitoring in heart failure reflects the right heart's preload status and gives insight into fluid status. Elevated CVP in HF patients often indicates fluid overload and can guide diuretic use to relieve symptoms.
2. **Pulmonary Capillary Wedge Pressure (PCWP)**: PCWP, obtained through a pulmonary artery catheter, represents left-sided filling pressures. Elevated PCWP is associated with pulmonary congestion and dyspnea in HF patients. Keeping PCWP within optimal ranges can help minimize fluid buildup in the lungs.
3. **Cardiac Output (CO) and Cardiac Index (CI)**: Low CO and CI values indicate reduced heart performance in HF patients. Interventions aim to optimize CO to improve tissue perfusion. Monitoring these values can also help titrate inotropes to maintain adequate perfusion.
4. **Systemic Vascular Resistance (SVR)**: HF often triggers compensatory vasoconstriction to maintain blood pressure, resulting in increased SVR. Monitoring SVR helps guide the use of vasodilators, which can reduce afterload and improve CO.
5. **Mixed Venous Oxygen Saturation (SvO2)**: SvO2 provides an indirect measure of tissue oxygenation and cardiac function. Low SvO2 indicates poor oxygen delivery relative to consumption, suggesting the need

for increased CO.

MONITORING TOOLS AND TECHNIQUES

1. **Invasive Hemodynamic Monitoring**: Invasive monitoring devices, such as pulmonary artery catheters, offer thorough hemodynamic data in cases of acute decompensated heart failure. These devices directly measure CO and pressure, which is helpful for patients whose hemodynamics are unstable.
2. **Non-Invasive Monitoring**: Methods like echocardiography, bioimpedance, and Doppler ultrasound are valuable for chronic heart failure monitoring, especially in outpatient settings. These tools allow clinicians to assess left ventricular ejection fraction (LVEF) and valvular function, key indicators of HF severity and progression.
3. **Implantable Monitoring Devices**: Advanced heart failure patients may benefit from implantable devices that continuously monitor hemodynamic parameters, such as pulmonary artery pressures, providing early warnings of fluid overload and reducing hospital readmissions.

THERAPEUTIC IMPLICATIONS OF HEMODYNAMIC MONITORING

- **Fluid Management**: Monitoring CVP and PCWP helps determine fluid overload status, guiding diuretic therapy to relieve symptoms of pulmonary and systemic congestion.
- **Optimizing Cardiac Output**: In patients with low CO, hemodynamic monitoring helps guide the use of inotropic agents to improve myocardial contractility, especially in acute settings.
- **Afterload Reduction**: Monitoring SVR assists in adjusting vasodilator therapies, which can reduce the workload on the heart and improve forward flow, especially in cases of high SVR.

Hemodynamic monitoring of HF patients offers crucial information for modifying treatment and enhancing quality of life. Physicians can minimize the risk of hospitalization, optimize cardiac function, and prevent HF exacerbations by constantly monitoring pressures, volume status, and cardiac performance.

HEMODYNAMIC CONSIDERATIONS IN POST-OPERATIVE CARE

Hemodynamic monitoring faces particular difficulties during post-operative treatment, particularly for patients who have had significant surgery or who already have heart issues. In order to prevent problems, promote recovery, and increase patient outcomes, hemodynamic stability is essential during the post-operative phase. Maintaining appropriate tissue perfusion, controlling fluid balance, and identifying early warning indicators of problems are all crucial monitoring goals during this stage.

Key Hemodynamic Goals in Post-Operative Care

1. **Maintaining Optimal Blood Pressure and Cardiac Output**: After surgery, patients often experience fluctuations in blood pressure and CO due to anesthesia, blood loss, and fluid shifts. Monitoring helps ensure these values remain within target ranges to support organ function, particularly for high-risk patients.
2. **Fluid Balance and Volume Status**: Surgical procedures, especially abdominal and cardiac surgeries, can lead to significant fluid shifts and blood loss. Accurate assessment of fluid status is essential to guide fluid replacement therapy, prevent fluid overload, and avoid complications like pulmonary edema. Parameters like CVP, PCWP, and urine output are particularly informative in guiding fluid management.

3. **Detecting Hypoperfusion and Hypoxemia**: Postoperative hypoperfusion, if left unchecked, can lead to tissue hypoxia and organ dysfunction. By monitoring parameters like MAP, SvO2, and lactate levels, clinicians can detect and address hypoperfusion early to prevent complications such as acute kidney injury (AKI) and respiratory failure.

TOOLS AND TECHNIQUES FOR POST-OPERATIVE HEMODYNAMIC MONITORING

1. **Invasive Monitoring**: In high-risk surgeries or patients with significant cardiovascular risk, invasive tools like arterial catheters and central venous lines provide real-time data on blood pressure, CVP, and oxygen saturation. These tools are particularly useful in managing hemodynamic instability.
2. **Non-Invasive Methods**: Techniques like Doppler ultrasound and pulse contour analysis offer continuous monitoring without the risks associated with invasive procedures. These methods are advantageous for stable patients or those in recovery following moderate-risk surgeries.
3. **Telemetry and Portable Monitoring**: In the post-surgical phase, especially for patients who are mobile, portable telemetry allows for continuous monitoring of heart rate, rhythm, and vital signs, enabling early detection of arrhythmias or hemodynamic compromise.

MANAGING COMMON HEMODYNAMIC ISSUES IN POST-OPERATIVE CARE

- **Hypotension**: Often due to hypovolemia, vasodilation from anesthesia, or blood loss. Treatment includes fluid resuscitation, vasopressors, or inotropes, guided by hemodynamic monitoring to avoid excessive or inadequate resuscitation.
- **Arrhythmias**: Post-operative arrhythmias, particularly atrial fibrillation, are common in cardiac and thoracic surgeries. Monitoring with telemetry or ECG helps detect arrhythmias promptly, allowing for interventions like electrolyte correction or pharmacologic management.
- **Pain and Anxiety**: Pain and anxiety can increase sympathetic nervous system activity, raising blood pressure and heart rate. Analgesia and sedation are essential not only for patient comfort but also to stabilize hemodynamic parameters.

Post-operative hemodynamic monitoring is vital to detect instability, manage fluid balance, and support optimal cardiac function. By implementing tailored monitoring strategies, healthcare teams can minimize complications, support recovery, and ultimately improve patient outcomes.

In managing diverse clinical scenarios, hemodynamic monitoring provides essential insights to guide patient care, detect early complications, and optimize interventions. This chapter explored specific applications of hemodynamic monitoring across critical situations, from managing hypotension and shock to addressing complex hemodynamic challenges in sepsis, heart failure, and post-operative care. Each scenario presents distinct hemodynamic patterns and risks, highlighting the need for a tailored, patient-centered approach.

Clinicians can use monitoring data to guide fluid and medication modifications, enhance patient stability, and proactively address potential issues by having a thorough understanding of these diverse hemodynamic profiles. Hemodynamic evaluations are essential to attaining the greatest results for patients, whether managing abrupt changes in blood pressure during shock, keeping an eye on cardiac function in heart failure, or guaranteeing a safe recovery following surgery. This information not only gives medical personnel the ability to react appropriately in emergency situations, but it also boosts their self-assurance and proficiency in providing high-quality care in a variety of clinical settings.

CHAPTER EIGHT

Fluid Management and Volume Resuscitation

Fluid management is foundational in critical care, where maintaining optimal blood volume and ensuring adequate organ perfusion can mean the difference between recovery and deterioration. Hemodynamic monitoring plays an essential role in fluid assessment, allowing clinicians to gauge a patient's fluid status and tailor interventions accordingly. In this chapter, we explore the nuanced strategies for assessing fluid requirements, conducting fluid challenges, and managing potential volume overload.

In order to make sure that every intervention is in line with the patient's particular physiological requirements, we first look at how hemodynamic measures can be used to evaluate fluid status. Next, we discuss the fluid challenge, a useful diagnostic technique to assess a patient's fluid responsiveness and inform resuscitation choices. In order to avoid consequences like pulmonary edema and organ failure, we conclude by going over methods for recognizing and treating volume overload, an often-ignored but crucial component of fluid treatment. The goal of this chapter is to give medical professionals evidence-based, hands-on techniques for fluid resuscitation so they may confidently and successfully manage fluid balance in critical care situations.

ASSESSING FLUID STATUS USING HEMODYNAMIC PARAMETER

Accurate assessment of fluid status is essential for guiding fluid management in critically ill patients, as both fluid deficits and overload can lead to severe complications. Hemodynamic parameters offer critical insights into a patient's volume status, guiding clinical decisions for resuscitation and maintenance therapy.

Key hemodynamic metrics commonly used for assessing fluid status include:

1. **Central Venous Pressure (CVP)**: Traditionally used to estimate right ventricular preload, CVP reflects the blood pressure in the thoracic vena cava near the right atrium. Although CVP alone may not precisely indicate overall fluid status, trends in CVP changes can provide valuable information about a patient's response to fluid administration or depletion.
2. **Pulmonary Capillary Wedge Pressure (PCWP)**: Measured using a pulmonary artery catheter, PCWP estimates left ventricular preload. Higher PCWP values generally indicate increased fluid levels in the pulmonary circuit, which may suggest volume overload, particularly in patients with heart failure or other cardiac complications.
3. **Stroke Volume Variation (SVV) and Pulse Pressure Variation (PPV)**: These dynamic parameters are highly responsive to changes in intravascular volume in

mechanically ventilated patients. High values of SVV or PPV often suggest that a patient is likely to benefit from fluid administration, making these measures useful for evaluating fluid responsiveness.

4. **Cardiac Output (CO) and Cardiac Index (CI)**: Cardiac output, adjusted for body size as cardiac index, reflects the amount of blood the heart pumps per minute. Assessing CO and CI alongside other parameters, like CVP and PCWP, provides a fuller picture of a patient's hemodynamic status and the potential need for fluid resuscitation.

5. **Ultrasound or Echocardiographic Assessment**: Point-of-care ultrasound has become increasingly valuable for evaluating fluid status. By assessing inferior vena cava (IVC) variability, left ventricular filling, and overall cardiac function, ultrasound provides non-invasive, real-time insights into volume status, especially in patients where invasive methods may pose risks.

Understanding all of these factors at once, in addition to the patient's clinical background, is necessary for an effective fluid assessment. Additionally, while using each parameter alone, clinicians need to be aware of its limits. For example, whereas CVP and PCWP offer baseline information on pulmonary and venous pressures, they are not very good at forecasting fluid responsiveness by themselves; instead, they are best understood in the context of the larger hemodynamic profile.

FLUID CHALLENGE: WHEN AND HOW

A diagnostic and therapeutic technique for determining a patient's fluid responsiveness is a fluid challenge. In order to maximize tissue perfusion without running the risk of fluid overload, this procedure assists physicians in determining whether giving a patient more fluids will enhance their cardiac output. Careful evaluation, the right timing, and knowledge of the patient's hemodynamic reaction to fluid delivery are necessary while doing a fluid challenge.

When to Perform a Fluid Challenge

Fluid challenges are commonly performed in patients with suspected hypovolemia or shock, where there is uncertainty about fluid status and whether the patient will benefit from additional volume. Key scenarios include:

- **Hypotension and Low Urine Output**: Patients exhibiting hypotension and decreased urine output may benefit from a fluid challenge to assess whether volume expansion will improve circulation.
- **Signs of Poor Perfusion**: Evidence of inadequate tissue perfusion, such as altered mental status, cool extremities, or elevated lactate levels, can indicate the need for a fluid challenge to boost cardiac output.
- **Shock States**: In cases of sepsis, cardiogenic, or distributive shock, fluid challenges are often necessary to stabilize hemodynamics and support perfusion, particularly when dynamic assessments indicate fluid responsiveness.

How to Perform a Fluid Challenge

1. **Baseline Measurement**: Begin by measuring baseline hemodynamic parameters, such as stroke volume, cardiac output, and blood pressure. These values serve as a reference for assessing the patient's response to the fluid challenge.
2. **Administering Fluid Bolus**: Typically, a fluid bolus of 250–500 mL of isotonic crystalloid (e.g., saline) is administered over 10–15 minutes. This volume and rate may vary based on patient characteristics, such as cardiac function and comorbidities.
3. **Monitoring Response**: Following the bolus, reassess the hemodynamic parameters. A positive response generally involves a 10–15% increase in stroke volume or cardiac output. The patient's response is also evaluated by improved blood pressure, urine output, and clinical signs of perfusion.
4. **Evaluation and Decision-Making**: If the patient reacts favorably, more fluids could be suggested to enhance perfusion even further, as long as there are no dangers of fluid overload. Alternative therapies, including vasopressors, should be explored if there is no discernible change in hemodynamics. The patient may not be fluid-responsive.

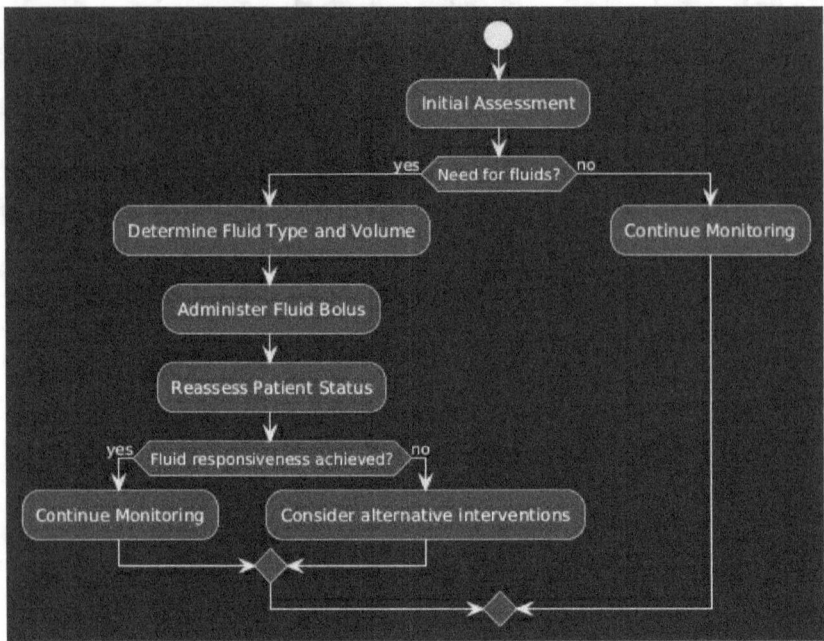

Fig 8.1: A flowchart summarizing the steps of the fluid challenge process

VOLUME OVERLOAD: DETECTION AND MANAGEMENT

Volume overload occurs when there is an excessive accumulation of fluid in the body, often resulting in complications such as pulmonary edema, heart failure exacerbations, and compromised tissue perfusion. In critically ill patients, especially those undergoing aggressive fluid resuscitation, the risk of volume overload is significant, making it crucial to detect and manage early to avoid adverse outcomes.

Detecting Volume Overload

1. **Physical Examination**: Clinical signs include edema, jugular venous distention (JVD), pulmonary crackles, and increased weight. Rapid weight gain, especially over 24–48 hours, may indicate fluid retention.
2. **Hemodynamic Parameters**:
   - **Central Venous Pressure (CVP)** and **Pulmonary Artery Pressure (PAP)**: Elevated CVP or PAP can indicate fluid accumulation, particularly in patients with compromised cardiac function.
   - **Stroke Volume Variability (SVV)**: In patients receiving mechanical ventilation, SVV can help gauge fluid responsiveness and identify overload.
3. **Imaging and Laboratory Tests**:
   - **Chest X-Ray or Lung Ultrasound**: Can reveal pulmonary congestion or pleural effusion.
   - **B-type Natriuretic Peptide (BNP) Levels**: Elevated BNP is often associated with volume overload in heart

failure patients, as it reflects increased cardiac wall stretch.

MANAGEMENT OF VOLUME OVERLOAD

1. **Diuretic Therapy**:
- **Loop Diuretics** (e.g., furosemide): Commonly used to promote renal excretion of sodium and water, decreasing fluid volume effectively.
- **Combination Diuretic Therapy**: Adding thiazide diuretics can enhance efficacy in patients resistant to loop diuretics alone.
2. **Renal Replacement Therapy (RRT)**:
- **Hemodialysis or Ultrafiltration**: Used in severe cases where conventional diuretics fail or the patient is in renal failure. Ultrafiltration allows for gradual removal of fluid to reduce overload without drastic electrolyte changes.
3. **Fluid Restriction**:
- **Limiting Fluid Intake**: Particularly important in patients with heart or renal failure. Restricting oral and IV fluids can help manage and prevent further fluid accumulation.
4. **Hemodynamic Monitoring and Adjustment**:
- **Titration of Vasopressors and Inotropes**: Adjusting medications that affect cardiac output and vascular tone can help manage fluid overload by reducing venous return and afterload.
- **Close Monitoring of Hemodynamic Changes**: Ensuring that volume removal aligns with improvements in perfusion markers and symptoms without exacerbating hypotension or other complications.

Fluid management and volume resuscitation are vital in critical care, where maintaining the correct fluid balance can mean the difference between recovery and further complications. A structured approach—beginning with accurate assessment of fluid status through hemodynamic parameters, applying targeted fluid challenges, and vigilant monitoring for signs of volume overload—ensures that each patient receives tailored, effective care. Through understanding and managing fluid balance, healthcare providers can help optimize cardiovascular stability and tissue perfusion, which is essential in the successful management of critically ill patients. This chapter has underscored the importance of using comprehensive and precise strategies, highlighting how essential tools like hemodynamic monitoring, judicious use of fluids, and awareness of potential volume overload equip clinicians with the insights needed to make well-informed, impactful decisions at the bedside.

CHAPTER NINE

Pharmacology for Hemodynamic Management

Pharmacological agents play a fundamental role in hemodynamic management, providing critical support in stabilizing and optimizing cardiovascular function in patients facing acute illness or unstable conditions. This chapter covers key drug classes such as inotropes, vasopressors, and vasodilators, exploring their mechanisms, clinical applications, and appropriate contexts for use. Each category of drugs serves a unique purpose: inotropes help strengthen cardiac contraction, vasopressors improve blood pressure through vasoconstriction, and vasodilators manage hypertension by promoting vessel relaxation. Proper drug selection, dosage adjustment, and a thorough understanding of potential side effects are crucial for effective, safe management. This chapter also provides practical guidance on using these agents for common hemodynamic challenges, emphasizing the importance of individualized dosing and vigilant monitoring to achieve optimal outcomes.

INOTROPES, VASOPRESSORS, AND VASODILATORS EXPLAINED

In managing critically ill patients with hemodynamic instability, inotropes, vasopressors, and vasodilators are essential pharmacological agents. Each drug class affects cardiovascular function in specific ways, addressing different underlying issues related to cardiac output, blood pressure, and vascular tone. A thorough understanding of these drugs allows for tailored treatment in clinical scenarios such as shock, heart failure, and severe hypertension.

1. Inotropes

Drugs known as inotropes alter the contractility of the heart. They fall into one of two groups: positive inotropes, which make heartbeats stronger, or negative inotropes, which make them weaker. Since increasing cardiac output can enhance tissue perfusion and oxygenation, positive inotropes are especially helpful in heart failure and cardiogenic shock.

Mechanism of Action: Positive inotropes work primarily by increasing intracellular calcium in the myocardial cells, which strengthens contraction. Commonly used agents include dobutamine, dopamine, and milrinone.

Dobutamine acts mainly on beta-1 adrenergic receptors, enhancing myocardial contractility and slightly increasing heart rate, making it useful in heart failure without significantly raising systemic vascular resistance.

Dopamine at moderate doses also increases heart

contractility, but it has dose-dependent effects that can cause vasoconstriction at higher doses, which might be desirable or avoided depending on the clinical situation.

Milrinone, a phosphodiesterase-3 inhibitor, increases cardiac contractility by inhibiting cAMP breakdown, leading to increased intracellular calcium. It also has vasodilatory effects, reducing afterload and potentially improving cardiac output.

Clinical Application: Positive inotropes are indicated in situations where cardiac output is insufficient to meet metabolic demands, such as in acute heart failure or cardiogenic shock. Their use requires careful monitoring of cardiac output, systemic vascular resistance, and potential side effects like arrhythmias.

2. Vasopressors

Drugs known as vasopressors cause vasoconstriction, which raises blood pressure and systemic vascular resistance (SVR). They play a crucial role in treating hypotension, especially in shock situations where maintaining blood pressure is necessary to keep important organs perfused.

Mechanism of Action: Vasopressors stimulate alpha-adrenergic receptors on vascular smooth muscle, leading to vasoconstriction. Some agents also act on beta-adrenergic receptors, contributing to increased cardiac output. Examples include norepinephrine, epinephrine, phenylephrine, and vasopressin.

Norepinephrine is often the first-line vasopressor in septic shock due to its strong alpha-adrenergic activity with some beta-adrenergic effects, increasing both SVR and, to a lesser extent, cardiac output.

Epinephrine has potent effects on both alpha and beta receptors, increasing blood pressure and cardiac output, but it may increase lactate levels and myocardial oxygen demand.

Phenylephrine is a pure alpha-adrenergic agonist, making it effective for vasoconstriction without affecting heart rate significantly. It is useful when tachycardia limits the use of other vasopressors.

Vasopressin, a non-catecholamine vasoconstrictor, works on V1 receptors in vascular smooth muscle. It is often used as an adjunct to other vasopressors in septic shock, particularly when catecholamine doses are high.

Clinical Application: Vasopressors are critical in managing different types of shock, particularly septic, neurogenic, and anaphylactic shock. Careful titration is essential to avoid excessive vasoconstriction, which can impair tissue perfusion and lead to complications like limb ischemia or excessive cardiac workload.

3. Vasodilators

Vasodilators are used to reduce afterload and preload by relaxing vascular smooth muscle, resulting in vasodilation. This class of drugs is beneficial in conditions where reducing systemic or pulmonary vascular resistance can alleviate the heart's workload, such as in hypertensive emergencies and heart failure.

Mechanism of Action: Vasodilators can act on arterial, venous, or both vascular beds. Agents like nitroglycerin primarily dilate veins, reducing preload, while others like nitroprusside cause both arterial and venous dilation, lowering afterload and preload.

Nitroglycerin releases nitric oxide, which activates guanylate cyclase in vascular smooth muscle, causing vasodilation. It is particularly effective in reducing myocardial oxygen demand in ischemic heart disease. Nitroprusside also works via nitric oxide release and is a potent arterial and venous dilator, often used in hypertensive crises or severe heart failure. However, prolonged use requires caution due to potential cyanide toxicity.

Hydralazine specifically dilates arterioles, lowering afterload and is sometimes used in heart failure when beta-blockers or ACE inhibitors are contraindicated.

Clinical Application: Vasodilators are commonly indicated in hypertensive crises, heart failure, and certain forms of cardiogenic shock where reducing vascular resistance can improve cardiac output and tissue perfusion. Monitoring is necessary to prevent hypotension, reflex tachycardia, and, in some cases, cyanide toxicity with drugs like nitroprusside.

Inotropes, vasopressors, and vasodilators each serve a distinct function in the management of hemodynamic instability. Their roles often overlap, and the choice of drug and dosage depend on the specific hemodynamic parameters that need adjustment, patient comorbidities, and potential side effects. Optimal use of these drugs requires continuous monitoring, careful titration, and knowledge of each agent's pharmacodynamics to maximize therapeutic effects while minimizing risks.

PHARMACOLOGIC INTERVENTIONS FOR COMMON HEMODYNAMIC ISSUES

Hemodynamic instability can arise from various conditions, such as shock, heart failure, and hypertensive crises, each requiring specific pharmacologic interventions to stabilize cardiovascular function. Interventions often involve the use of inotropes, vasopressors, vasodilators, and anti-arrhythmic drugs, each with tailored roles in optimizing cardiac output, blood pressure, and tissue perfusion.

1. Shock Management

Pharmacologic intervention is frequently necessary to restore blood pressure and tissue perfusion in shock, regardless of whether it is septic, hypovolemic, or cardiogenic. Because they have strong vasoconstrictive effects that assist raise blood pressure and systemic vascular resistance (SVR), vasopressors like norepinephrine and dopamine are frequently used as first-line treatments in septic and distributive shock. Because it affects both alpha and beta receptors, epinephrine can be added or substituted in situations that call for both enhanced cardiac output and vascular resistance. Dobutamine and other inotropic medications are recommended for individuals in cardiogenic shock because they can improve cardiac output and myocardial contractility without causing severe vasoconstriction, which eases the strain on the failing heart.

2. Heart Failure

Pharmacologic therapy of acute or decompensated heart failure is to improve cardiac contractility and decrease preload and afterload. Important inotropes that improve cardiac contractility and can lessen pulmonary congestion are milrinone and dobutamine. Concurrent administration of diuretics, such as furosemide, is frequently used to lessen fluid overload, lower preload, and relieve fluid retention symptoms. In certain situations, vasodilators like nitroglycerin or nitroprusside are used to lower preload and afterload, increasing cardiac efficiency and lessening the strain on the heart.

3. Hypertensive Emergencies

Hypertensive crises often require immediate pharmacologic intervention to reduce blood pressure and prevent organ damage. Nitroprusside and labetalol are commonly used in emergencies, providing rapid blood pressure reduction while minimizing the risk of hypotension when carefully titrated. Calcium channel blockers like nicardipine are also effective, particularly in cases where peripheral vasodilation is required without significant reduction in cardiac output. For patients at risk of reflex tachycardia, beta-blockers such as esmolol may be added to control heart rate.

4. Arrhythmias and Cardiac Output Management

For hemodynamic instability due to arrhythmias, anti-arrhythmic drugs like amiodarone (for ventricular tachycardia or atrial fibrillation) are used to restore rhythm and stabilize cardiac output. Beta-blockers or calcium channel blockers may also be employed to control the heart rate in atrial fibrillation, which can improve hemodynamic stability by allowing for better ventricular filling and cardiac output.

Pharmacologic interventions for hemodynamic issues are crucial for managing conditions like shock, heart failure, hypertensive emergencies, and arrhythmias. By understanding the specific actions and indications of each drug class, clinicians can tailor interventions to the underlying pathophysiology, providing effective treatment that balances efficacy with safety. Continuous monitoring is essential to adapt dosages and avoid adverse effects, ensuring optimal outcomes for hemodynamically unstable patients.

DRUG DOSING CONSIDERATIONS AND SIDE EFFECTS

When using pharmacologic agents for hemodynamic management, appropriate dosing and awareness of side effects are critical to ensure both efficacy and patient safety. Hemodynamic drugs, such as **inotropes**, **vasopressors**, and **vasodilators**, can vary in their effects based on factors such as the patient's underlying condition, drug pharmacokinetics, and route of administration. Understanding dosing intricacies and monitoring for adverse effects are essential for clinicians to achieve therapeutic goals without exacerbating side effects.

1. Dosing Considerations

- **Patient-Specific Factors:** Dosing often requires adjustment based on patient-specific factors like age, weight, renal and hepatic function, and comorbidities. For example, in older patients, reduced renal or liver function may affect drug metabolism, necessitating lower doses or slower titration rates.
- **Titration and Therapeutic Goals:** Many hemodynamic drugs, especially vasopressors and inotropes, require careful titration to achieve specific hemodynamic targets such as blood pressure, cardiac output, or systemic vascular resistance. This titration allows clinicians to incrementally increase or decrease the dose while closely monitoring the patient's response.
- **Drug-Drug Interactions:** Hemodynamic drugs can interact with other medications, altering their efficacy and safety

profiles. For instance, beta-blockers can blunt the response to inotropes like dobutamine, while co-administration of vasodilators and diuretics may increase the risk of hypotension.
- **Dosing Based on Administration Route:** Many hemodynamic agents require intravenous (IV) administration due to rapid onset and predictable absorption. IV drugs are more controlled than oral forms, but improper IV administration can increase side effects. Central venous administration, preferred for drugs like norepinephrine and epinephrine, reduces the risk of extravasation but requires technical proficiency.

2. Side Effects by Drug Class

- **Inotropes (e.g., Dobutamine, Milrinone):**
  → **Common Side Effects:** Tachycardia, arrhythmias, hypotension, and increased myocardial oxygen demand.
  → **Specific Considerations:** Dobutamine, commonly used in heart failure, can cause dose-dependent tachycardia and arrhythmias, especially in patients with ischemic heart disease. Milrinone, a phosphodiesterase inhibitor, also increases heart rate but can cause hypotension due to its vasodilatory effect.
- **Vasopressors (e.g., Norepinephrine, Epinephrine, Dopamine):**
  → **Common Side Effects:** Hypertension, tachycardia, peripheral ischemia, and arrhythmias.
  → **Specific Considerations:** Norepinephrine is a first-line vasopressor in septic shock due to its strong alpha-adrenergic effects, which increase vascular resistance and blood pressure. However, it can cause peripheral vasoconstriction leading to ischemia, especially in high doses or prolonged use.

Epinephrine, while also effective, has a higher risk of tachyarrhythmias and hyperglycemia due to its beta-adrenergic activity.

- **Vasodilators (e.g., Nitroglycerin, Nitroprusside):**
  → **Common Side Effects:** Hypotension, reflex tachycardia, and in some cases, cyanide toxicity.
  → **Specific Considerations:** Nitroprusside, used for rapid blood pressure control, releases cyanide as a byproduct. Prolonged infusions, especially in patients with renal impairment, can lead to cyanide toxicity, presenting as metabolic acidosis and altered mental status. Nitroglycerin is safer but can cause significant hypotension and reflex tachycardia, particularly if titrated too quickly.
- **Antiarrhythmics (e.g., Amiodarone, Lidocaine):**
  → **Common Side Effects:** Bradycardia, hypotension, and in the case of amiodarone, potential pulmonary toxicity and thyroid dysfunction.
  → **Specific Considerations:** Amiodarone, often used in atrial and ventricular arrhythmias, requires careful monitoring due to its potential for pulmonary fibrosis with long-term use. Both lidocaine and amiodarone can depress cardiac output in patients with low ejection fractions.

3. Monitoring and Managing Side Effects

- **Regular Monitoring:** Continuous monitoring of hemodynamic parameters (e.g., blood pressure, heart rate, oxygen saturation) is essential for adjusting doses and detecting adverse effects early.
- **Proactive Management:** In the case of arrhythmias induced by inotropes, adding beta-blockers or reducing the inotrope dose may help control heart rate. For vasodilators causing hypotension, reducing the infusion rate or co-administering fluids can mitigate hypotensive effects.

- **Patient Education:** Educating patients on potential side effects (if they are awake and alert) and involving them in their care can improve symptom reporting and timely management of adverse reactions.

When it comes to hemodynamic pharmacology, cautious dosage and side effect management are essential. Clinicians can customize treatment to meet the specific needs of each patient, proactively monitor for side effects, and modify therapies to preserve hemodynamic stability and avoid complications by being aware of the pharmacodynamics and pharmacokinetics of each medicine.

Pharmacologic management of hemodynamic instability in critical care requires a deep understanding of inotropes, vasopressors, vasodilators, and other drug classes. Each of these agents comes with unique properties that impact cardiac function, vascular tone, and overall patient stability. Knowing when and how to utilize these drugs can significantly influence patient outcomes, particularly in acute situations such as shock, heart failure, and sepsis.

The importance of precise dosing, close monitoring, and awareness of potential side effects cannot be overstated. Proper dosing minimizes adverse effects, and vigilant monitoring allows clinicians to adjust therapy dynamically in response to the patient's hemodynamic profile. Furthermore, understanding the clinical situation and context of each pharmacologic intervention—whether it be improving cardiac output or stabilizing blood pressure—helps guarantee that treatments are both efficient and targeted.

The intricate, multidimensional strategy required for safe and efficient pharmacologic hemodynamic management has been emphasized in this chapter, highlighting the crucial role that these medications play in helping clinicians support patients who are in critical condition.

CHAPTER TEN

Hemodynamic Case Studies and Clinical Application

In clinical practice, hemodynamic monitoring moves beyond theoretical concepts and into critical decision-making that directly impacts patient outcomes. Real-world application of hemodynamic principles requires the integration of knowledge, technical skill, and sound clinical judgment, all of which are essential for managing patients in dynamic and complex situations.

In order to demonstrate how hemodynamic principles can be applied in various contexts, this chapter provides a number of case studies that evolve from straightforward to more intricate situations. To assist therapists in converting theoretical knowledge into practical insights, each case study offers a detailed explanation of assessment, critical thinking, and intervention techniques. We will also discuss typical mistakes that can jeopardize patient care, like misinterpreting hemodynamic data or relying too much on one parameter, and how to prevent them.

By examining these cases, clinicians can strengthen their ability to solve complex hemodynamic challenges with confidence and skill. This chapter aims to reinforce critical thinking pathways, support sound decision-making, and improve the quality of patient-centered care in hemodynamic monitoring.

REAL-WORLD CASE STUDIES: FROM SIMPLE TO COMPLEX

In the clinical setting, the real challenge in hemodynamic monitoring is not only in understanding the data but also in making timely, precise decisions based on the complexities each unique patient scenario presents. Using real-world case studies helps bridge theoretical knowledge and clinical practice, providing insights into the application of hemodynamic monitoring in patient care. This section will delve into case studies from basic to complex, illustrating essential hemodynamic assessments, decision pathways, and interventions for various clinical conditions.

Simple Case Study: Hypotension Management in Postoperative Patients

One of the most straightforward applications of hemodynamic monitoring is in postoperative hypotension management. In these cases, understanding the baseline hemodynamic status of the patient is critical. Imagine a case of a patient recovering from abdominal surgery presenting with low blood pressure.

In this scenario, the clinician may start with basic hemodynamic monitoring, focusing on mean arterial pressure (MAP) and central venous pressure (CVP). Low MAP with normal CVP could indicate low vascular resistance, suggesting vasodilation as a result of anesthesia or surgical stress. Treatment might begin with volume resuscitation to ensure the patient is not volume-depleted, followed by low-dose vasopressors if hypotension persists. This straightforward case allows for hands-on application of basic hemodynamic principles.

Intermediate Case Study: Sepsis-Induced Cardiovascular Collapse

Managing a patient in septic shock involves more complex monitoring and interventions. Sepsis causes profound vasodilation and capillary leak, resulting in decreased systemic vascular resistance (SVR) and hypovolemia. A hemodynamic assessment of a septic patient might reveal low MAP, low CVP, and decreased stroke volume.

In this case, fluid resuscitation is initially performed to counteract hypovolemia, with CVP monitoring guiding the volume status. Persistent hypotension despite adequate volume resuscitation would prompt the use of vasopressors, such as norepinephrine, to increase SVR and MAP. Advanced hemodynamic monitoring, such as assessing stroke volume variation or cardiac output, can further refine treatment by optimizing fluid and drug therapy, a practice crucial in managing such multifaceted conditions.

Complex Case Study: Cardiogenic Shock Post-Myocardial Infarction

A patient in cardiogenic shock following a myocardial infarction (MI) presents one of the most challenging scenarios for hemodynamic monitoring. This condition is marked by inadequate cardiac output and tissue perfusion, despite a high filling pressure in the left ventricle, often leading to pulmonary congestion and respiratory distress.

In this complex case, the clinician must monitor pulmonary capillary wedge pressure (PCWP) and cardiac index (CI) to assess left ventricular function. High PCWP with low CI suggests a failing left ventricle, a hallmark of cardiogenic shock. Interventions would typically involve inotropic agents, such as dobutamine, to support cardiac output, along with diuretics or ultrafiltration to reduce pulmonary congestion. In severe cases, mechanical circulatory support (e.g., intra-aortic balloon pump or extracorporeal membrane oxygenation) may be necessary. This level of hemodynamic management requires a deep understanding of cardiac function and precise interpretation of invasive parameters.

CRITICAL REFLECTION ON CASE STUDY APPLICATION

These case studies show that hemodynamic monitoring is a dynamic aspect of patient care that supports clinical decision-making, not just a tool for observation. In straightforward situations, it facilitates rapid evaluations and timely interventions; in more complicated situations, it offers in-depth understanding of pathophysiology that permits highly customized interventions. Clinicians can improve patient outcomes, improve therapy approaches, and better predict consequences by researching these cases.

In addition to strengthening technical proficiency, real-world case studies develop critical thinking skills and the capacity to make quick decisions based on a thorough comprehension of each patient's particular hemodynamic profile.

CRITICAL THINKING AND DECISION-MAKING PATHWAYS

In hemodynamic management, effective critical thinking and decision-making pathways are essential as they enable clinicians to synthesize complex data and deliver timely interventions. Mastering these skills is crucial in settings where a patient's hemodynamic status can rapidly change, as in critical care, cardiology, or emergency medicine. Critical thinking here involves systematic assessment, understanding complex physiological relationships, and recognizing patterns that inform timely and effective clinical decisions.

Developing a Structured Approach to Decision-Making

Structured decision-making models, such as the Systematic Processing Model and the Hypothetico-Deductive Model, offer frameworks that facilitate logical thinking in hemodynamic monitoring. These models advise medical professionals to begin with a general comprehension of a patient's symptoms and work their way down to specifics:

1. **Hypothetico-Deductive Reasoning**: This approach involves creating potential hypotheses based on initial patient data and progressively narrowing down the possibilities as new information arises. For instance, if a patient presents with low blood pressure, potential causes could range from hypovolemia to cardiogenic shock. Through sequential testing (e.g., checking central venous pressure or cardiac output), the clinician can confirm or rule out each cause until

the diagnosis is clear.

2. **Systematic Processing**: This model involves analyzing patient data methodically, considering each piece of information individually before integrating it into the larger picture. For example, in a hypotensive patient, clinicians may systematically assess preload, afterload, cardiac output, and systemic vascular resistance, each contributing to the larger hemodynamic profile. This process enables a comprehensive assessment that minimizes the risk of overlooking key data.

Key Components of Decision-Making in Hemodynamic Management

1. **Pattern Recognition**: Experienced clinicians can often recognize patterns that indicate specific hemodynamic conditions, such as fluid overload or shock states. Pattern recognition relies heavily on clinical experience and knowledge of normal versus abnormal waveforms, trends, and parameter ranges.

2. **Prioritization and Rapid Response**: In critical care, clinicians must rapidly prioritize interventions to address life-threatening conditions. This requires both speed and accuracy. For example, in cases of cardiogenic shock, immediate inotropic support may be prioritized to sustain cardiac output before addressing underlying etiologies.

3. **Dynamic Reassessment**: Hemodynamic parameters are not static; they can fluctuate in response to interventions or changes in the patient's condition. Effective decision-making requires frequent reassessment of hemodynamic data post-intervention, such as following a fluid challenge or vasopressor administration. This dynamic approach helps avoid under- or over-treatment and allows for adjustments based on real-time data.

4. **Risk-Benefit Analysis**: Clinicians frequently have to weigh the advantages and disadvantages of various therapy approaches. Vasopressors, for example, can improve perfusion when used to raise blood pressure in septic shock, but they also raise the risk of tissue ischemia because they cause severe vasoconstriction. A crucial component of safe, efficient hemodynamic regulation is weighing the trade-offs.

Applying Critical Thinking in Complex Scenarios

In practice, decision-making pathways are not linear and often involve multiple steps of reassessment and adjustment. For example:

- **Case of Septic Shock**: A patient presents with hypotension and signs of septic shock. The clinician initiates fluid resuscitation but must monitor central venous pressure and MAP to gauge fluid responsiveness. If blood pressure remains low, the next step may be to introduce a vasopressor like norepinephrine while continuously reassessing hemodynamic data to avoid tissue ischemia.
- **Case of Heart Failure with Hypotension**: Treating hypotension in heart failure patients is complex due to the risk of fluid overload. The clinician may use cardiac index (CI) and pulmonary capillary wedge pressure (PCWP) to determine the need for inotropic support or diuretics, balancing the need for adequate cardiac output against the risk of exacerbating heart failure symptoms.

Avoiding Common Pitfalls

A systematic decision-making process also helps clinicians avoid common pitfalls, such as confirmation bias (favoring data that supports an initial assumption), anchoring (relying too heavily on initial information), and over-reliance on technology without clinical correlation. Regular practice, reflection, and collaboration can help clinicians refine their critical thinking skills, allowing them to navigate complex clinical scenarios effectively.

In hemodynamic management, critical thinking and structured decision-making are vital in providing high-quality care. A clinician's ability to interpret data dynamically, assess risks, and make prompt, informed decisions can significantly impact patient outcomes, particularly in critical care environments where hemodynamic instability can escalate quickly.

COMMON PITFALLS AND HOW TO AVOID THEM IN HEMODYNAMIC MONITORING AND MANAGEMENT

Hemodynamic monitoring and management are critical in the care of patients in high-acuity settings, but they come with specific challenges and common pitfalls. Avoiding these pitfalls requires knowledge, attentiveness, and adherence to best practices. Below are some of the most frequently encountered pitfalls in hemodynamic monitoring, along with strategies to prevent them.

1. Misinterpretation of Hemodynamic Data

Misinterpreting data is one of the most prevalent issues in hemodynamic monitoring. It can occur when clinicians over-rely on single parameters or when they fail to consider the physiological context of the readings. For example, solely depending on central venous pressure (CVP) to assess fluid status can lead to inappropriate fluid management, as CVP may not accurately reflect intravascular volume in all patients.

How to Avoid:
- Use a comprehensive approach that includes multiple parameters (e.g., cardiac output, mean arterial pressure, and systemic vascular resistance) rather than focusing on a single metric.
- Train regularly in data interpretation and familiarize

yourself with normal ranges and common causes of aberrant readings.
- Consider the patient's entire clinical picture, including recent interventions and underlying health conditions, to accurately contextualize data.

2. Inadequate Calibration and Zeroing of Equipment

Accurate measurements from hemodynamic monitoring equipment require proper zeroing and calibration. Either not calibrating and zeroing transducers or doing so incorrectly are frequent mistakes. Data may get biased as a result, which could lead to inappropriate treatment choices.

How to Avoid:

- Follow standard protocols to calibrate and zero equipment at the start of each shift and any time the patient's position changes.
- Place the transducer at the level of the right atrium (phlebostatic axis) to maintain consistency.
- Regularly check equipment functionality, especially if readings seem inconsistent with the clinical presentation.

3. Failure to Recognize and Correct for Artifacts

Movement, electrical interference, or incorrect line positioning are common causes of artifacts, which can skew results. For instance, catheter kinks or tube length may dampen or amplify arterial line waveforms, resulting in inaccurate pressure readings.

How to Avoid:

- Routinely inspect waveforms for signs of artifacts and evaluate if readings align with the patient's clinical status.
- Troubleshoot line placement, check for kinks, and minimize excess tubing. Replace lines if necessary.
- Implement strategies such as reducing patient movement and using equipment with built-in filters for electrical

noise.

4. Over-Reliance on Technology Without Clinical Correlation

Technology in hemodynamic monitoring can provide critical insights, but a common pitfall is to rely on it without correlating the data with clinical observations. This can result in "automation bias," where clinicians trust device readings without critical evaluation, even when those readings may not match the patient's symptoms.

How to Avoid:

- Continuously assess patients physically and cross-reference clinical symptoms with monitor data.
- Encourage team members to report discrepancies between clinical findings and monitor outputs to ensure a comprehensive evaluation.
- Engage in regular training that emphasizes integrating technology with hands-on assessment to maintain a balanced approach.

5. Delayed Response to Hemodynamic Changes

A delayed response to changes in hemodynamic status can occur due to task overload, misinterpretation of data, or lack of established protocols for certain conditions. For example, a patient with septic shock may experience a sudden drop in blood pressure, and failure to initiate vasopressor therapy quickly can lead to severe complications.

How to Avoid:

- Implement standardized protocols and algorithms to guide rapid responses for specific hemodynamic changes, such as hypotension or tachycardia.
- Designate roles within the healthcare team to monitor trends and alert providers when critical changes occur.
- Encourage regular simulation training to improve response time and ensure that all team members

understand their roles in high-stakes scenarios.

6. Inadequate Understanding of Pharmacologic Interventions

When hemodynamic support drugs like vasopressors, inotropes, or vasodilators are used, there's a risk of improper dosing or misuse if the clinician is not fully aware of the pharmacologic effects. Administering too high a dose of a vasopressor, for example, can lead to tissue ischemia, while underdosing may fail to stabilize blood pressure adequately.

How to Avoid:

- Keep up-to-date with training on the pharmacology of drugs used in hemodynamic management and always double-check dosing guidelines.
- Assess the patient's entire hemodynamic profile and adjust drug dosages in small increments, allowing time to observe effects before increasing.
- Use decision-support tools or consult with a pharmacist for complex medication regimens, especially for patients with multiple comorbidities.

7. Lack of Communication and Coordination in the Care Team

Miscommunication or lack of coordination among team members can lead to errors, such as duplicative interventions or missed opportunities for timely treatment. This can be particularly problematic during patient handoffs or when managing patients who require complex hemodynamic interventions.

How to Avoid:

- Implement standardized communication protocols like SBAR (Situation, Background, Assessment, Recommendation) during patient handoffs to ensure consistency.
- Use checklists for high-risk procedures and engage in daily huddles to synchronize care plans among the

multidisciplinary team.
- Encourage an open culture where all team members feel empowered to ask questions and clarify orders if needed.

8. Failure to Monitor Trends Over Time

A single hemodynamic measurement is often less valuable than understanding how parameters trend over time. Clinicians sometimes overlook trends and focus instead on momentary values, potentially missing early signs of deterioration or improvement.

How to Avoid:

- Regularly review trends in parameters like blood pressure, heart rate, and cardiac output instead of relying solely on snapshot readings.
- Use graphical displays on monitors to visualize parameter trends over time, helping to identify gradual changes that may require intervention.
- Ensure proper documentation of key hemodynamic parameters, especially during critical events, to create a comprehensive patient history that informs future decisions.

9. Neglecting the Influence of Comorbidities on Hemodynamic Interpretation

Comorbid conditions like chronic heart failure, renal dysfunction, or chronic hypertension can alter baseline hemodynamic values, making standard ranges less applicable. This pitfall often leads to either overestimating or underestimating the severity of a hemodynamic alteration.

How to Avoid:

- Take a thorough patient history and adjust baseline expectations based on pre-existing conditions.
- Collaborate with specialists when managing patients with complex comorbidities, ensuring that adjustments to

hemodynamic goals are appropriate.
- Use individualized monitoring strategies for patients with chronic conditions that deviate from typical norms, recognizing that these individuals may require tailored interventions.

It takes a combination of technical proficiency, clinical knowledge, and proactive communication to avoid hemodynamic monitoring errors. In order to optimize outcomes for critically ill patients, clinicians who are alert, knowledgeable, and eager to learn new things are better able to deliver high-quality hemodynamic treatment.

CHAPTER ELEVEN

Quick Reference Guides and Cheat Sheets

The complexity of hemodynamic monitoring and management in critical care requires clinicians to have access to precise and immediate information. Quick reference guides and cheat sheets serve as essential tools, providing a condensed source of critical data for healthcare professionals. These guides streamline access to information on normal hemodynamic values, troubleshooting steps, and medication dosing recommendations, facilitating rapid clinical decision-making.

Many non-invasive techniques for hemodynamic monitoring are now accessible thanks to recent developments in medical technology, which eliminate the need for invasive catheterization and give thorough, real-time cardiovascular data. These methods provide quicker and safer evaluations, which is particularly helpful for patients who are at high risk for intrusive monitoring or in outpatient settings. Some of the most popular cutting-edge non-invasive procedures will be discussed here.

NORMAL HEMODYNAMIC VALUES AND RANGES: DETAILED GUIDE

Accurate interpretation of hemodynamic parameters is essential in managing critically ill patients. Having a clear understanding of normal hemodynamic values helps clinicians detect deviations that may indicate underlying pathology or response to treatment. Below is a detailed guide to key hemodynamic measurements and their normal ranges, including explanations to aid in understanding each parameter's role in clinical assessments.

1. Central Venous Pressure (CVP)

- **Normal Range:** 2–6 mmHg (can vary slightly depending on specific clinical settings)
- **Significance:** CVP reflects the pressure within the thoracic vena cava near the right atrium. It provides insights into right ventricular preload and, indirectly, the volume status of a patient. Low CVP may indicate hypovolemia, while high CVP often suggests right heart dysfunction or fluid overload.

2. Mean Arterial Pressure (MAP)

- **Normal Range:** 70–100 mmHg
- **Significance:** MAP represents the average arterial pressure throughout a cardiac cycle and is a key determinant of organ perfusion. Maintaining MAP within normal limits is crucial for adequate tissue perfusion. Values below 65 mmHg may suggest compromised blood flow to organs,

while values above 100 mmHg could indicate hypertension or increased systemic vascular resistance (SVR).

3. Cardiac Output (CO)

- **Normal Range:** 4–8 L/min
- **Significance:** Cardiac output is the total volume of blood the heart pumps per minute. It's calculated as the product of heart rate (HR) and stroke volume (SV). Low CO may indicate heart failure or hypovolemia, whereas high CO could result from fever, sepsis, or hyperthyroidism.

4. Cardiac Index (CI)

- **Normal Range:** 2.5–4.0 L/min/m²
- **Significance:** Cardiac index adjusts cardiac output to body surface area (BSA), providing a more individualized measure of cardiac function. It is particularly useful in patients of varying body sizes. Low CI often suggests inadequate cardiac function for a patient's specific metabolic needs.

5. Stroke Volume (SV)

- **Normal Range:** 60–100 mL/beat
- **Significance:** Stroke volume is the amount of blood ejected from the left ventricle with each heartbeat. It is affected by preload, afterload, and contractility. Low stroke volume may indicate heart failure, hypovolemia, or increased afterload, while high SV may be present in hyperdynamic states.

6. Pulmonary Artery Pressure (PAP)

- **Normal Range:** Systolic 15–30 mmHg, Diastolic 4–12 mmHg
- **Significance:** PAP is measured through a pulmonary artery catheter and provides information about the pressure in the pulmonary artery, reflecting the right heart's function and the pulmonary vascular resistance. Elevated PAP may

suggest pulmonary hypertension, left heart dysfunction, or volume overload.

7. Pulmonary Capillary Wedge Pressure (PCWP)

- **Normal Range:** 6–12 mmHg
- **Significance:** PCWP is an estimate of left atrial pressure and is used to assess left ventricular preload. Elevated PCWP is often indicative of left heart failure or volume overload, while low PCWP can signal hypovolemia.

8. Systemic Vascular Resistance (SVR)

- **Normal Range:** 800–1200 dynes·sec·cm^{-5}
- **Significance:** SVR reflects the resistance the left ventricle must overcome to circulate blood through the systemic circulation. It's calculated based on MAP, CO, and CVP. Increased SVR often occurs in vasoconstriction or shock states, while decreased SVR can be seen in vasodilation, sepsis, or anaphylaxis.

9. Pulmonary Vascular Resistance (PVR)

- **Normal Range:** 100–250 dynes·sec·cm^{-5}
- **Significance:** PVR represents the resistance in the pulmonary circulation. Elevated PVR is associated with conditions like pulmonary hypertension or acute respiratory distress syndrome (ARDS), and it challenges the right ventricle to maintain adequate blood flow.

10. Oxygen Delivery (DO$_2$)

- **Normal Range:** 900–1100 mL/min
- **Significance:** Oxygen delivery is the amount of oxygen transported to tissues per minute. It's calculated based on CO and arterial oxygen content. Inadequate DO$_2$ may indicate impaired perfusion and oxygenation, leading to tissue hypoxia.

Summary Table Idea:

A table summarizing these values and parameters can serve as a quick reference in the clinical setting. It could look something like this:

Parameter	Normal Range	Clinical Significance
Central Venous Pressure (CVP)	2–6 mmHg	Indicates volume status and right heart function
Mean Arterial Pressure (MAP)	70–100 mmHg	Key determinant of organ perfusion
Cardiac Output (CO)	4–8 L/min	Reflects overall cardiac performance
Cardiac Index (CI)	2.5–4.0 L/min/m²	Adjusted CO based on body surface area
Stroke Volume (SV)	60–100 mL/beat	Volume ejected per beat, impacted by preload, afterload, and contractility
Pulmonary Artery Pressure (PAP)	15–30 mmHg systolic; 4–12 mmHg diastolic	Reflects pulmonary pressure
Pulmonary Capillary Wedge Pressure (PCWP)	6–12 mmHg	Indicates left heart function and volume status
Systemic Vascular Resistance (SVR)	800–1200 dynes·sec·cm^{-5}	Resistance against left ventricular ejection
Pulmonary Vascular Resistance (PVR)	100–250 dynes·sec·cm^{-5}	Right ventricular resistance
Oxygen Delivery	900–1100 mL/min	Amount of oxygen

| (DO₂) | | delivered to tissues |

These numbers provide a starting point for clinical evaluation, assisting in determining whether a patient's hemodynamic condition is within normal bounds or necessitates treatment.

QUICK TROUBLESHOOTING FOR EQUIPMENT ISSUES

Effective hemodynamic monitoring relies heavily on the accurate functioning of equipment, including catheters, transducers, monitors, and tubing. Equipment-related issues can result in inaccurate readings, leading to potential misinterpretations. Here is a comprehensive troubleshooting guide covering common equipment problems and quick solutions.

1. Line Occlusion or Kinking

- **Symptoms**: Zero readings, dampened waveform, or fluctuating pressures.
- **Troubleshooting Steps**:
    - Inspect the catheter tubing and connections to identify visible kinks or bends.
    - Ensure all connections are tight and secure to prevent disruptions in pressure transmission.
    - Flush the line using a pressurized saline flush system to clear potential blockages.
    - If occlusion persists, consider repositioning the catheter or replacing the tubing.

2. Air Bubbles in the Line

- **Symptoms**: Erratic waveform readings or dampened signals.
- **Troubleshooting Steps**:
    - Inspect the entire tubing for air bubbles, as even small bubbles can interfere with accurate readings.
    - Remove air bubbles by tapping the line gently while

flushing to push air out.
- If the bubble is in the transducer, disconnect the tubing from the patient, clear the air, and then reconnect.
- Maintain the system's pressure bag at 300 mmHg to minimize the risk of air entering the system.

3. Incorrect Zeroing of Transducer

- **Symptoms**: Off-baseline readings, incorrect pressure values.
- **Troubleshooting Steps**:
  - Confirm the transducer is leveled at the phlebostatic axis (4th intercostal space at the mid-axillary line) to ensure accurate pressure readings.
  - Re-zero the transducer by closing the stopcock to the patient, opening it to air, and pressing the "zero" function on the monitor.
  - If readings still appear incorrect, repeat the zeroing process, ensuring the stopcock setup is correct.

4. Dampened or Exaggerated Waveforms

- **Symptoms**: Waveforms either show reduced amplitude (dampened) or excessive peaks (exaggerated).
- **Troubleshooting Steps**:
  - Check for the presence of blood clots or debris within the catheter or tubing. Flush the line if safe and necessary.
  - Assess the tubing length; if it is excessively long, it may dampen the signal.
  - Verify the system is free from excessive stopcocks or unnecessary connectors, as these can interfere with signal transmission.
  - Confirm that all elements of the monitoring setup, including transducer and tubing, are designed

for hemodynamic monitoring, as incompatible components can distort waveforms.

5. Incorrect Calibration of Equipment

- **Symptoms**: Consistently inaccurate or drifting pressure readings.
- **Troubleshooting Steps**:
    - Recalibrate the transducer by ensuring it is exposed to air and verifying it reads zero before reconnecting to the patient.
    - For advanced monitoring systems, use the device's specific calibration method as outlined by the manufacturer.
    - Check that calibration occurs periodically throughout a shift, particularly after position changes, to maintain accuracy.

6. Fluctuating Pressure Bag or Saline Flush System Issues

- **Symptoms**: Absence of waveform or dampened trace due to improper flow or pressure.
- **Troubleshooting Steps**:
    - Verify that the pressure bag is inflated to 300 mmHg to maintain adequate flow within the system.
    - Ensure the saline flush bag has not depleted, as this can disrupt the continuous flow and cause dampened signals.
    - If the flush device malfunctions, replace it with a new flush system to restore adequate flow.

7. Transducer Over- or Under-Damping

- **Symptoms**: Overdamping leads to sluggish waveforms; underdamping results in overly spiked waveforms.
- **Troubleshooting Steps**:
    - Evaluate the catheter for blood clots or air, as these can lead to overdamping. Clear the line or replace the catheter if necessary.

- If the waveform is spiking, verify that the system's tubing is rigid enough for hemodynamic monitoring, as flexible or kinked tubing may cause issues.
- Perform a "fast flush" test by quickly flushing saline through the system to observe oscillation patterns, which can reveal damping issues that need correction.

8. Electrical or Signal Interference

- **Symptoms**: Unstable or erratic readings, which may not correlate with the patient's clinical status.
- **Troubleshooting Steps**:
  - Minimize surrounding electronic equipment that may cause interference, or use dedicated lines and equipment designed to shield from electrical interference.
  - Ensure cables are properly grounded and securely connected to avoid signal disruption.
  - Check for damaged wires or connectors and replace them if damaged.

Summary Checklist

For quick access, here's a checklist to maintain equipment accuracy:

- **Inspect connections and tubing** regularly for occlusions, air bubbles, and leaks.
- **Zero and level the transducer** at the beginning of monitoring and after each patient repositioning.
- **Maintain pressure in the flush system** to prevent interruptions.
- **Clear air bubbles** promptly to avoid signal dampening.
- **Perform calibration checks** periodically throughout monitoring.

Frequent equipment maintenance and inspection will significantly lower hemodynamic reading mistakes and guarantee that the clinical data gathered accurately depicts the patient's physiological condition.

MEDICATION DOSING CHARTS FOR HEMODYNAMIC AGENTS

Medication dosing charts for hemodynamic agents are essential tools for clinicians managing acute hemodynamic instability. They provide quick reference dosing, routes of administration, titration guidance, and safety considerations for key pharmacologic agents used in critical care. Here's an overview of essential hemodynamic agents, including **inotropes**, **vasopressors**, and **vasodilators**, along with dosing information that aligns with clinical standards.

1. Inotropes

Inotropes are used to enhance cardiac contractility, typically in patients with low cardiac output or compromised myocardial function.

- **Dobutamine**:
    - **Initial Dose**: 2-5 mcg/kg/min via continuous IV infusion.
    - **Titration**: Increase by 2-3 mcg/kg/min every 10-15 minutes as needed.
    - **Max Dose**: Typically up to 20 mcg/kg/min.
    - **Considerations**: Monitor for tachyarrhythmias; indicated primarily in low cardiac output states without severe hypotension.
- **Milrinone**:
    - **Loading Dose**: 50 mcg/kg IV over 10 minutes (optional).
    - **Maintenance Dose**: 0.375-0.75 mcg/kg/min IV

infusion.
- **Considerations**: Renal clearance requires dose adjustment in renal impairment; risk of arrhythmias and hypotension.

2. Vasopressors

The fundamental purpose of vasopressors is to keep the perfusion pressure in hypotensive shock at a suitable level.

- **Norepinephrine**:
  - **Initial Dose**: 0.01-0.5 mcg/kg/min, adjusted based on response.
  - **Titration**: Increase by 0.02-0.05 mcg/kg/min increments.
  - **Max Dose**: Up to 3 mcg/kg/min in extreme cases.
  - **Considerations**: First-line vasopressor for septic shock; caution with prolonged use due to risk of tissue ischemia.
- **Epinephrine**:
  - **Initial Dose**: 0.01-0.5 mcg/kg/min.
  - **Titration**: Adjust in increments of 0.01-0.1 mcg/kg/min.
  - **Max Dose**: Up to 1 mcg/kg/min, depending on clinical scenario.
  - **Considerations**: Used as a second-line vasopressor or in anaphylactic shock; side effects include tachycardia and increased myocardial oxygen demand.
- **Vasopressin**:
  - **Dose**: Typically 0.03 units/min IV infusion (not titrated).
  - **Considerations**: Often used as an adjunct to norepinephrine in septic shock; avoid bolus dosing due to risks of coronary and peripheral ischemia.

3. Vasodilators

Vasodilators are used to lower pulmonary or systemic vascular resistance, usually in heart failure or hypertension with high afterload.

- **Nitroglycerin**:
  - **Initial Dose**: 5-10 mcg/min IV infusion.
  - **Titration**: Increase by 5-10 mcg/min every 5-10 minutes as tolerated.
  - **Max Dose**: Up to 200 mcg/min for refractory cases.
  - **Considerations**: Monitor blood pressure closely; avoid in patients with hypotension or those on PDE inhibitors.
- **Sodium Nitroprusside**:
  - **Initial Dose**: 0.3-0.5 mcg/kg/min.
  - **Titration**: Increase by 0.5 mcg/kg/min as needed.
  - **Max Dose**: Up to 10 mcg/kg/min, with close monitoring due to risk of cyanide toxicity.
  - **Considerations**: Rapid onset; used in hypertensive emergencies but requires caution for prolonged use.

Key Considerations for Safe Dosing

- **Continuous Monitoring**: Blood pressure, heart rate, and other hemodynamic parameters should be monitored continuously to assess drug efficacy and avoid adverse effects.
- **Dose Titration**: Adjustments should be made based on patient response and tolerance, with frequent reassessment.
- **Organ Function**: Liver and kidney function should be evaluated regularly, as certain drugs (like milrinone) are renally cleared and may require dose adjustments in renal impairment.
- **Side Effect Profile**: Awareness of the unique side effects of each agent—such as cyanide toxicity with nitroprusside or arrhythmias with inotropes—is crucial.

The purpose of this dosing guide is to ensure the safe and efficient management of hemodynamic disturbances by offering prompt, evidence-based insights that are in line with best practices in critical care pharmacology. When using these agents, always refer to the specific patient consideration and institutional protocols.

Cheat sheets and quick reference guides are essential tools for successful and efficient hemodynamic management in critical care settings. Essential resources have been gathered in this chapter to help clinicians with hemodynamic value assessment, equipment troubleshooting, and precise medicine dosage. These materials help to improve patient outcomes and decision-making by giving quick access to standard ranges, troubleshooting techniques, and exact dose instructions. In the end, a clinician's capacity to react quickly and effectively to intricate hemodynamic scenarios can be improved by keeping a solid basis in these quick-reference tools, which will benefit patient safety and professional confidence.

CHAPTER TWELVE
Frequently Asked Questions

This chapter covers some of the most frequent queries and misunderstandings that physicians and hemodynamic monitoring novices run into. Even seasoned clinicians frequently ask for clarification on technical elements, clinical applications, and best practices because hemodynamic monitoring can be a complicated practice. From comprehending the complexities of equipment to analyzing certain measurements, these inquiries offer crucial information to boost competence and confidence.

Alongside these answers, this chapter offers expert tips for those new to the field, sharing advice to help streamline workflows, enhance accuracy, and support patient care in high-stakes environments. Whether troubleshooting or fine-tuning techniques, this FAQ section aims to serve as a reliable resource for navigating the complexities of hemodynamic monitoring with clarity and precision.

ADDRESSING COMMON CONCERNS AND MISCONCEPTIONS

There are many myths and worries about hemodynamic monitoring, especially for medical professionals trying to strike a balance between efficient monitoring and patient comfort and safety. We discuss some of the most frequent queries and misconceptions in the subject here:

1. **Concern: Hemodynamic Monitoring is Too Complex for New Clinicians** Many clinicians feel overwhelmed by the perceived complexity of hemodynamic monitoring, especially when confronted with a range of parameters and equipment. However, starting with fundamental concepts—like understanding the key parameters (e.g., preload, afterload, and cardiac output)—can provide a solid foundation, building confidence over time. Breaking down the learning process into manageable steps can make these complex concepts easier to understand and apply.

2. **Misconception: Monitoring is Only Necessary for Critically Ill Patients** While critical care settings are where hemodynamic monitoring is often emphasized, it's also essential in other situations, such as post-surgery or with patients at risk of fluid imbalances. Routine monitoring can be invaluable in early detection of issues before they progress, allowing for timely intervention and improved patient outcomes.

3. **Concern: Invasive Monitoring is Always the Best Choice for Accuracy** Although invasive methods such

as arterial lines provide precise measurements, they're not always necessary and can increase the risk of complications like infections. Non-invasive options, such as Doppler ultrasound or pulse contour analysis, have proven effective in many situations, offering a safe alternative with sufficient accuracy, especially in stable patients or routine monitoring.

4. **Misconception: All Devices are Calibrated the Same Way** Different equipment may need different calibration methods and procedures, which, if not followed correctly, may result in readings that differ. Periodic equipment inspections and routine calibration in accordance with manufacturer instructions can assist guarantee accurate data capture. Errors due to miscalibration can also be avoided with proper equipment training.

5. **Concern: Interpreting Abnormal Readings Quickly is Challenging** When it comes to sudden changes in readings, clinicians often worry about making rapid, accurate interpretations. Using quick reference guides, such as those included in Chapter 11, and having a solid understanding of typical hemodynamic patterns can improve response time and help clinicians make timely adjustments. Training and familiarity with both normal and abnormal waveforms, as covered in Chapter 4, further assist in quick, reliable interpretation.

6. **Misconception: Hemodynamic Monitoring Only Focuses on the Heart** While cardiac parameters are central to hemodynamic monitoring, it's also essential to understand the role of the vascular system and the impact of peripheral resistance. Parameters like systemic vascular resistance (SVR) and pulmonary vascular resistance (PVR) offer insight into the broader circulatory system, aiding in comprehensive patient assessment.

These commonly expressed worries and misconceptions emphasize the value of ongoing education and real-world experience. By addressing them head-on, physicians can employ hemodynamic monitoring technologies more confidently and efficiently, which improves patient safety and care.

EXPERT TIPS FOR BEGINNERS IN HEMODYNAMIC MONITORING

Hemodynamic monitoring is an essential skill in critical care, and while it can initially feel overwhelming, there are several key strategies to help beginners become comfortable and proficient. Here are some expert tips that can serve as a foundation for building confidence and competence:

1. **Master the Basics of Key Parameters**
   Start with a solid understanding of essential hemodynamic parameters, such as cardiac output, blood pressure, stroke volume, and vascular resistance. Knowing what these values indicate about a patient's condition is fundamental. Recognize the significance of each parameter and how it correlates with physiological processes to interpret readings accurately.

2. **Familiarize Yourself with Monitoring Devices**
   Equipment can vary significantly, so it's essential to become familiar with the devices and monitors commonly used in your setting. Learn the specific functions, calibration processes, and potential error messages associated with each device. Practicing with the equipment in a non-emergency setting, if possible, can help reduce errors and improve response time in real situations.

3. **Emphasize Safety and Infection Control**

Procedures like arterial line insertion and central venous catheterization carry a risk of infection and complications. Strict adherence to aseptic technique, monitoring for signs of infection, and routinely inspecting the insertion site are critical for patient safety. Beginners should be vigilant in following protocols to maintain sterility and should seek guidance if any questions arise regarding infection control.

4. **Develop Interpretation Skills through Patterns**

   Interpreting data involves understanding normal and abnormal patterns rather than isolated readings. Familiarize yourself with typical waveforms and trends associated with different clinical scenarios, such as shock or heart failure, to build a mental library of expected responses and deviations. Comparing patterns over time can provide insight into patient trends and responses to interventions.

5. **Don't Ignore Non-Invasive Options**

   Non-invasive techniques, such as Doppler ultrasound and pulse contour analysis, offer valuable insights without the risks associated with invasive methods. Especially for beginners, these options can provide essential information with minimal risk, allowing you to gather data while you gain experience with more complex monitoring.

6. **Stay Calm and Use Critical Thinking During Emergencies**

   In high-stakes environments, it's common to feel pressured to make quick decisions. Take a moment to gather the necessary data, analyze it, and verify before proceeding. Remember, quick reactions are less important than accurate assessments. Relying on basic principles and established protocols helps ensure that actions are grounded in best practices.

7. **Seek Mentorship and Collaborate with Experienced**

Clinicians

Learning from experienced colleagues is invaluable for beginners in hemodynamic monitoring. Observing techniques, discussing case studies, and asking for feedback can accelerate your learning process. Experienced team members can provide practical insights and share tips that may not be found in textbooks or training manuals.

8. **Use Reference Guides and Cheat Sheets**

   Keeping handy reference materials, such as normal hemodynamic values, common troubleshooting tips, and quick charts on drug dosages (covered in previous chapters), can be incredibly helpful. These can serve as a guide when you're still familiarizing yourself with frequent clinical scenarios and responses.

9. **Document and Reflect on Each Experience**

   Each monitoring session provides valuable learning experiences, whether through the complexity of a case, a challenge in interpreting data, or a technical issue with equipment. Documenting these cases and reflecting on them allows you to track your progress, solidify learning points, and identify areas for further growth.

Different equipment may need different calibration methods and procedures, which, if not followed correctly, may result in readings that differ. Periodic equipment inspections and routine calibration in accordance with manufacturer instructions can assist guarantee accurate data capture. Errors due to miscalibration can also be avoided with proper equipment training.

In hemodynamic monitoring, understanding the underlying principles and addressing common questions and misconceptions is vital to improving patient outcomes and building clinician confidence. This chapter has clarified frequent areas of uncertainty and provided foundational knowledge and practical tips for beginners. By acknowledging common challenges and offering solutions, we emphasize the importance of ongoing learning, reflection, and adaptation in the dynamic field of hemodynamic monitoring.

The professional advice provided in this chapter helps novice practitioners improve their abilities and ability to make decisions. Overall, technical expertise alone is not enough for good hemodynamic monitoring; critical thinking, teamwork, and ongoing skill development are also necessary. By focusing on these fundamentals, practitioners can help provide safer, more efficient patient care in a variety of clinical settings.

CONCLUSION

We have examined the foundations of hemodynamic monitoring in this book, covering everything from key ideas and equipment use to clinical uses and medication interventions. The goal of each chapter has been to develop a thorough understanding by offering both theoretical knowledge and useful skills that may be used immediately in patient care. Effective hemodynamic monitoring and patient care are based on critical factors like preload, afterload, cardiac output, and vascular resistance, as well as the significance of waveforms, equipment calibration, and efficient troubleshooting.

SUMMARY OF KEY CONCEPTS

1. **Understanding Hemodynamics**: Core concepts like cardiac output, preload, afterload, and vascular resistance shape our understanding of cardiovascular health and the effects of therapeutic interventions.
2. **Monitoring Tools and Techniques**: Both invasive and non-invasive methods offer unique insights, each suited to specific clinical scenarios and patient needs.
3. **Critical Decision-Making**: Analyzing hemodynamic data and interpreting waveforms requires critical thinking, especially in dynamic or high-risk situations like shock and heart failure.
4. **Pharmacologic Management**: In-depth knowledge of inotropes, vasopressors, and vasodilators, as well as their effects on hemodynamics, equips clinicians to tailor therapies accurately.
5. **Case Applications and Troubleshooting**: Real-life applications and troubleshooting skills help practitioners navigate challenges and make informed decisions in acute care settings.

ADDITIONAL RESOURCES FOR CONTINUED LEARNING

To further expand your understanding, consider exploring additional resources such as specialized textbooks, peer-reviewed journals, and online courses. These resources offer updates on evolving hemodynamic technologies, case studies, and new clinical guidelines that enhance decision-making in diverse patient scenarios.

- **Textbooks**: Look for specialized hemodynamic and critical care textbooks.
- **Peer-reviewed Journals**: Journals like *Critical Care Medicine* and *Journal of Cardiovascular Nursing* publish studies and reviews on the latest advances in hemodynamic monitoring.
- **Online Courses and Certifications**: Platforms like Coursera, Medscape, and AACN offer courses on advanced hemodynamic monitoring and critical care techniques.

BOOKS AND GUIDES

- "The Heart Disease Prevention Cookbook" by Sarah Stewart
  This book offers a collection of heart-healthy recipes and nutritional advice to help you maintain a balanced diet that supports cardiovascular health.

- "Prevent and Reverse Heart Disease: The Revolutionary, Scientifically Proven, Nutrition-Based Cure" by Caldwell B. Esselstyn Jr., M.D.
  A comprehensive guide to dietary approaches for preventing and reversing heart disease, supported by scientific research.

- "The Cardiovascular Cure: How to Strengthen Your Self-Defense Against Heart Disease and Stroke" by John P. Cooke and Judith Zimmer
  This book provides insights into improving cardiovascular health through lifestyle changes and understanding the latest research.

- "Mastering ECG EKG Interpretation: A Comprehensive Guide for Beginners: ECG Interpretation Made Easy" by Joan Hampton
  A beginner-friendly book that simplifies ECG interpretation, making it accessible for students, healthcare professionals, and ideal for healthcare providers who interpret ECGs regularly. Buy on Amazon

- "ECG/EKG and Cardiac Conditions: Interpreting Key Disease Patterns"
  This guide focuses on noting key ECG/EKG signs of heart conditions, making it easier to interpret these patterns

for all levels of healthcare professionals. Buy on Amazon

Interested in furthering your knowledge in Hemodynamic Monitoring?

If you are keen to advance your skills and gain practical, hands-on experience, we encourage you to reach out to greenwayorg1@gmail.com. By using the coupon code HEMO24, you can enjoy a 10% discount on all training courses. Don't miss out on the opportunity to enhance your expertise in this critical area of healthcare.

Contact us today and take your learning to the next level!

HOW TO APPLY WHAT YOU'VE LEARNED TO REAL-WORLD PRACTICE

The skills and knowledge gained from this guide will serve as a valuable foundation in clinical practice. Practitioners should aim to integrate this information gradually, focusing on the nuances of interpreting hemodynamic data within the context of patient-specific variables. Embrace collaborative learning environments, seek mentorship from seasoned practitioners, and actively participate in discussions on patient care strategies. Remember that experience, paired with ongoing learning, is key to mastering hemodynamic monitoring and providing the best possible care for patients.

APPENDICES

The appendices offer additional tools, resources, and reference material to further support your application of hemodynamic monitoring knowledge. These sections provide quick-access reference materials for bedside practice, common calculations, and essential terminology.

Appendix A: Hemodynamic Monitoring Checklist

This checklist serves as a practical guide for setting up and performing hemodynamic monitoring, ensuring that all steps are completed accurately and safely. Key elements include:

- **Pre-Monitoring Preparation**: Confirming patient identifiers, obtaining informed consent, and gathering all necessary supplies.
- **Equipment Setup**: Calibrating equipment, verifying monitor settings, and establishing baseline readings.
- **Monitoring Protocols**: Documenting initial and continuous data, checking line patency, and ensuring sterile technique throughout.
- **Safety Checks**: Regular assessments of alarms, troubleshooting, and periodic reassessment of insertion sites to prevent infection or displacement.

This checklist can be printed and used as a reminder for safe and effective hemodynamic monitoring.

Appendix B: Hemodynamic Formulas and Calculations

This appendix includes commonly used formulas to calculate key hemodynamic parameters, providing a quick reference for clinicians. Some essential formulas covered:

- **Cardiac Output (CO)**: CO = SV × HR where SV is stroke volume and HR is heart rate.
- **Systemic Vascular Resistance (SVR)**: SVR = MAP−CVP/CO x 80 where MAP is mean arterial pressure and CVP is central venous pressure.
- **Pulmonary Vascular Resistance (PVR)**: PVR = MPAP −PCWP/CO×80 where MPAP is mean pulmonary arterial pressure and PCWP is pulmonary capillary wedge pressure.

These formulas help convert raw data into meaningful clinical insights, assisting in real-time decision-making at the bedside.

Appendix C: Glossary of Hemodynamic Terms

A glossary of terms provides definitions and explanations of essential hemodynamic vocabulary, ideal for quick reference. Key terms include:

- **Afterload**: The resistance the left ventricle must overcome to circulate blood.
- **Preload**: The initial stretching of the cardiac myocytes prior to contraction, commonly influenced by venous return.
- **Contractility**: The intrinsic strength of cardiac muscle contraction, independent of preload and afterload.
- **Mean Arterial Pressure (MAP)**: The average arterial pressure during a single cardiac cycle, crucial for assessing organ perfusion.

This glossary ensures clarity on terminology, promoting effective communication and understanding among healthcare team members.

THE END

www.ingramcontent.com/pod-product-compliance
Lightning Source LLC
Chambersburg PA
CBHW071454220526
45472CB00003B/801